Thanks for all of your great help! Best wishes and luck in your future career.

Autopsy in the 21st Century

Jody E. Hooper • Alex K. Williamson
Editors

Autopsy in the 21st Century

Best Practices and Future Directions

Springer

Editors
Jody E. Hooper
Department of Pathology
Johns Hopkins University
Baltimore, MD
USA

Alex K. Williamson
Department of Pathology & Laboratory
Medicine, Zucker School of Medicine
at Hofstra / Northwell
Hempstead, NY
USA

ISBN 978-3-319-98372-1 ISBN 978-3-319-98373-8 (eBook)
https://doi.org/10.1007/978-3-319-98373-8

Library of Congress Control Number: 2018962268

This Springer imprint is published by the registered company Springer Nature Switzerland AG
The registered company address is: Gewerbestrasse 11, 6330 Cham, Switzerland

To my parents, Professor Paul and Mrs. Pam Hooper, with deepest gratitude – JEH

To my daughter, Juliet Maven, for inspiring me to work toward a better tomorrow – AKW

Preface

Every 5 years or so, another paper is published reaffirming the continuing clinical value of the autopsy in uncovering unsuspected clinical diagnoses, many of which could, if treated, have altered the course of the patient's care. It is somewhat intriguing that there appears to be a need to continue to "make the case" for the existence of the autopsy on a relatively regular basis. There is, of course, the pervasive sense among clinical colleagues that modern diagnostic techniques are so advanced that patients no longer die with undiagnosed or misdiagnosed disease – yet the data clearly and consistently show otherwise. In many settings, pathologists also continue to shy away from this important clinical activity. As practice models have begun to focus on physician productivity and directly link that to compensation, the time it takes to do an autopsy well is viewed as time away from RVU-generating activities. Training of future pathologists in the performance of autopsies has also come under examination. As the volume of the material pathology residents need to learn during their relatively short training period continues to grow (e.g., molecular pathology, informatics, whole slide imaging, *in vivo* microscopy, participation in patient safety initiatives), program directors are looking for ways to make space in the schedule for these growing areas, and it has been suggested that perhaps the 50 autopsy requirement to sit for the board examination in anatomic pathology needs to be reconsidered.

Despite these "attacks" on seemingly multiple fronts, the autopsy remains the cornerstone of quality assurance in medicine. The 2015 Institute of Medicine report "Improving Diagnosis in Heath Care" identifies postmortem examination as a key data source for detecting and monitoring diagnostic errors and further encourages (Recommendation 4C) that the Department of Health and Human Services provide funding for this medical procedure. The Autopsy Working Group of the Association of Pathology Chairs has also recently endorsed the importance of maintaining autopsy instruction as a key component of pathology residency training, recommends that the current minimum requirement of 50 autopsies not be reduced (at this time), and further urges such programs to have a dedicated Autopsy Service Director to assure adequate instruction in autopsy techniques. This stance is based on the simple reality that the autopsy continues to fulfill an important diagnostic role in the current practice of medicine. As new treatments become available, use of the autopsy remains vital in assessing the effectiveness and consequences of those therapies. For example, much of what we are learning about the side effects of the new immunotherapies has come from autopsy investigations.

But the autopsy of today is not the same as it was even a decade ago. Ongoing evolution is clearly necessary to maintain the utility and value of the autopsy. New techniques are available to augment the traditional gross and microscopic examinations, and there is a greater call to use data obtained from autopsies for purposes beyond simply answering unanswered questions about individual cases. These "new frontiers" for the autopsy are a major focus of this book. Advanced imaging modalities and molecular testing are becoming routine components of the autopsy in many settings. The value of tissue, often rapidly obtained after death, is becoming increasingly appreciated both for research projects and for building annotated banks and repositories. Data collection, aggregation across cases, and analysis are now being used to advance the role for the autopsy in quality management and supporting efforts in population-based healthcare. Realizing this potential will require standardization in data collection and recording.

This book provides both a historical perspective on the autopsy and plots a path forward. It discusses ways to increase the value of the autopsy, both locally and on a larger scale. It addresses not only what the autopsy is, but what it could be. Any pathology department with an autopsy service should seriously consider the ideas developed in this book, based on the real experiences of the authors at their own institutions. Readers will undoubtedly find ways to improve autopsy practices at their own institutions.

New Haven, CT, USA John Sinard

Acknowledgment

Both Editors would like to acknowledge their joint mentor in postmortem care, Dr. Stephen Geller. Jody Hooper also recognizes Dr. Ralph Hruban and Dr. Angelo DeMarzo for their support and recognition of the value of autopsy. Alex Williamson would also like to acknowledge Dr. Charles Hirsch for his instruction and inspiration in caring for decedents and their families, as well as Dr. James Crawford for his championing the autopsy.

The Editors gratefully acknowledge the Johns Hopkins Pathology Photography Department, in particular Norm Barker, MS, MA, RBP, and Jon Christofersen, BA, MA, for their invaluable expertise and patience in contributing to the exhibits for this book.

Contents

Contributors

Gregory Chamberlin, MD Frank H. Netter MD School of Medicine at Quinnipiac University, North Haven, CT, USA

Kim A. Collins, MD Newberry Pathology Associates, Newberry, SC, USA

Sharing Hope South Carolina, Charleston, SC, USA

Eleonora Duregon, MD, PhD Department of Pathology, The Johns Hopkins University, Baltimore, MD, USA

Jun Fan, MD, PhD Department of Pathology, Stony Brook Medicine, Stony Brook, NY, USA

Billie Fyfe-Kirschner, MD Rutgers Robert Wood Johnson Medical School, Brunswick, NJ, USA

Stephen A. Geller, MD Department of Pathology and Laboratory Medicine, Weill Cornell Medical College, New York, NY, USA

Robert D. Hoffman, MD, PhD Department of Pathology, Microbiology and Immunology, Vanderbilt University Medical Center, Nashville, TN, USA

Jody E. Hooper, MD Department of Pathology, The Johns Hopkins University, Baltimore, MD, USA

Christine A. Iacobuzio-Donahue, MD, PhD Department of Pathology, David M. Rubenstein Center for Pancreatic Cancer Research, Human Oncology and Pathogenesis Program, Memorial Sloan Kettering Cancer Center, New York, NY, USA

Dylan V. Miller, MD Department of Pathology, University of Utah School of Medicine, Intermountain Medical Center, Murray, UT, USA

Harold Sanchez, MD, FCAP Frank H. Netter MD School of Medicine at Quinnipiac University, North Haven, CT, USA

Victor W. Weedn, MD, JD Department of Forensic Sciences, George Washington University, Washington, DC, USA

Alex K. Williamson, MD Department of Pathology & Laboratory Medicine, Zucker School of Medicine at Hofstra / Northwell, Hempstead, NY, USA

Part I

Introduction

A Short History of Human Dissection and the Autopsy

1

Stephen A. Geller

Introduction

The term "autopsy" implies "seeing for oneself" and derives from the Greek – *auto* for self and *opsy* for seeing – and, later, in Latin, as *autopsia*, "a seeing with one's own eyes" [1–14]. Originally used literally in the sense of self-examination or self-inspection by Galen, it later was employed to refer to an examination of "the body itself" [14]. Its application as the term for a postmortem examination of a human being (in animals, "necropsy" is generally employed) has been said to have been first used in the case of the Empress Feodorovna of Russia in 1829 [8, 14] although it was probably used as early as the sixteenth century in France (*autopsie*) and the seventeenth century in England, as shown in a 1651 portrait of two physicians, Charles Scarborough and Edward Arris, performing an autopsy [15]. Human dissections, driven by insatiable curiosity about human structure and disease, have been carried out for at least as long as recorded history.

The Development of Anatomy

No one knows when the actual first dissection of a human being for the purpose of obtaining knowledge took place. **Susruta**, in India during the Brahmin period, in approximately 5000 BCE, is the first person credited with performing such a procedure [1]. In **Babylonian times**, dissections on both humans and, especially, animals were performed, most likely only for the purpose of predicting the future. It is worth noting, however, that the Talmud of this time includes the first detailed listing of

S. A. Geller
Department of Pathology and Laboratory Medicine, Weill Cornell Medical College, New York, NY, USA

J. E. Hooper, A. K. Williamson (eds.), *Autopsy in the 21st Century*,
https://doi.org/10.1007/978-3-319-98373-8_1

human bones (Mishnah, Nid. 24b), the correct number of lobes of the human lung (Tomid 50a), and the structure of the esophagus (Hul. 43a) [2, 8, 16–18]. The Talmud also indicates that pig anatomy is similar to human anatomy (Ta'anit 21b) [8].

Early Greek and Roman Contributions

Homer (c. 900 BCE) and Hesiod (c. 750 BCE) each made a few anatomic observations, but the first person known to devote himself to the study of anatomy was **Alcmaeon** (c. 500 BCE), a native of the Greek colony of Croton in southern Italy; only a few fragments of his writings survive [1–3, 19, 20]. Pliny described **Herophilus** (335–280 BCE) [20], a student of the pragmatist Praxagoras of Cos (c. 400 BCE), as the "first man to search into the causes of disease" by human dissection. Herophilus described abdominal organs, the female genital tract, and the prostate gland, among other anatomic structures, and was the first to systematically study the brain and spinal cord [1]. By the third century BCE, dissection was practiced in Alexandria, Egypt, and both the Edwin Smith papyrus and the Ebers papyrus record a knowledge of anatomy [8].

Erasistratus of Chios (c. 310–250 BCE) recognized cirrhosis and the associated ascites. Son of a physician and disciple of the school of Cnidus, Erasistratus abandoned the humoral theory prevalent at the time and is the first physician recorded as performing what we would now call an autopsy: deliberately searching for the anatomic causes of pleurisy and pericarditis [1, 13].

Celsus (the first century), although probably not a physician, was a man of vast culture, well learned in the natural and medical sciences [1, 3]. He was one of the greatest contributors to medical knowledge, defining, among other things, the cardinal signs of inflammation. He may not have performed many human dissections himself but reportedly said, "…to open the bodies of the dead is necessary for learners…."

Galen of Pergamon (138–201) dissected the bodies of a few Roman gladiators and wrote about correlating the patient's signs and symptoms with a particular part of the body but performed most of his studies of anatomy on Barbary apes and pigs [1, 3, 8, 19]. The first to demonstrate arterial pulsations, the function of the recurrent laryngeal nerve [21], the function of the ureters, and other aspects of anatomy and physiology, Galen's writings on anatomy influenced and simultaneously impeded the development of medicine because of the contained dogmatic assertions based on animal anatomy, accepted almost universally for more than 13 centuries [22–25].

Dark Ages and Early Middle Ages

During the next approximately thousand years, there were isolated accounts of human dissections in Norway and Italy. A fourth-century fresco in a Christian cemetery in southeast Rome, uncovered in 1956, showing what appears to be the dissection of a woman's body, suggests that autopsies were condoned in early Christian times [26]. However, a tenth-century manuscript cites a physician friend of the Church Father Augustine as saying: “It pleased the ancient anatomists to examine the viscera of the dead to learn in what way they died, but for us *humanitas* prohibits this” [13, 27, 28]. In 1299, Pope Boniface VIII forbade the boiling of bodies to separate the flesh from the bones, a procedure performed to make it easier to bring the bones of crusaders back to Catholic burial grounds [8]. This may have led to the erroneous opinion that Catholicism does not allow autopsies. In the thirteenth century, the chronicle of the Franciscan monk Salimbene of Parma (1221–1290) alludes to a human dissection during the pestilence of 1286 [13]. Other isolated reports of dissections from that time exist and, during the renaissance, it is clear that they were allowed; a number of fourteenth- and fifteenth-century French, German, and Italian woodcuts are extant demonstrating human dissections in academic settings, with clear representation of teachers and students (Fig. 1.1) [8]. A number of Popes were autopsied, and Pope Sixtus IV (1471–1484) issued an edict permitting studies on human bodies by students at Bologna and Padua [8]. The first law authorizing autopsies was issued two centuries before by Frederick II (1194–1250), Emperor of the Holy Roman Empire [11].

Renaissance Contributions

In 1316 **Mondino de Luzzi** (Mundinus) (1270–1326) published a seminal anatomy textbook, *Anathomia*, which, in parts of Europe, became the primary source for learning about the structure of the human body (Fig. 1.2) [1–3, 8, 9]. This anatomical text, heavily influenced by Galen’s writings, was widely used until the sixteenth century. It is of interest that the frontispiece to *Anathomia* shows a young, long-haired prosector, perhaps representing **Alessandra Giliani** (1307–1326), the first known female anatomist who, in addition to assisting Mundinus and even correcting some Galenic concepts, developed a method for draining blood from the corpse and replacing it with colored dyes to better demonstrate arteries and veins [29–31].

Leonardo **Da Vinci**, in the fifteenth century, dissected many human bodies and may have been the one to first apply the term “coronary” to the cardiac vessels, likening them to a king’s crown [4]. Despite his extraordinary observational skills, Da Vinci was influenced by Galenic teachings. He described two autopsies, one performed on a hundred-year-old man who had died peacefully and the other on a child of 2 years, where “I found everything contrary to what it was in the case of the old man.” **Michelangelo** (1475–1564) also performed a few dissections, one of which he documented in a sketch, but his greatest interest was in surface anatomy.

In this period, autopsies were performed mostly on the bodies of criminals, but Alessandro **Benedetti** (1460–1525), who described gallstones, malrotation of the heart, and other entities, pointed to the necessity of performing autopsies on all people who died [24]. In 1507, Antonio **Benivieni** (1440–1502) published the first collection of autopsy reports. He was also the first physician known to have asked permission of relatives for performance of an autopsy, and his attempts to make clinical-pathologic correlations may have set the stage for Morgagni. Although

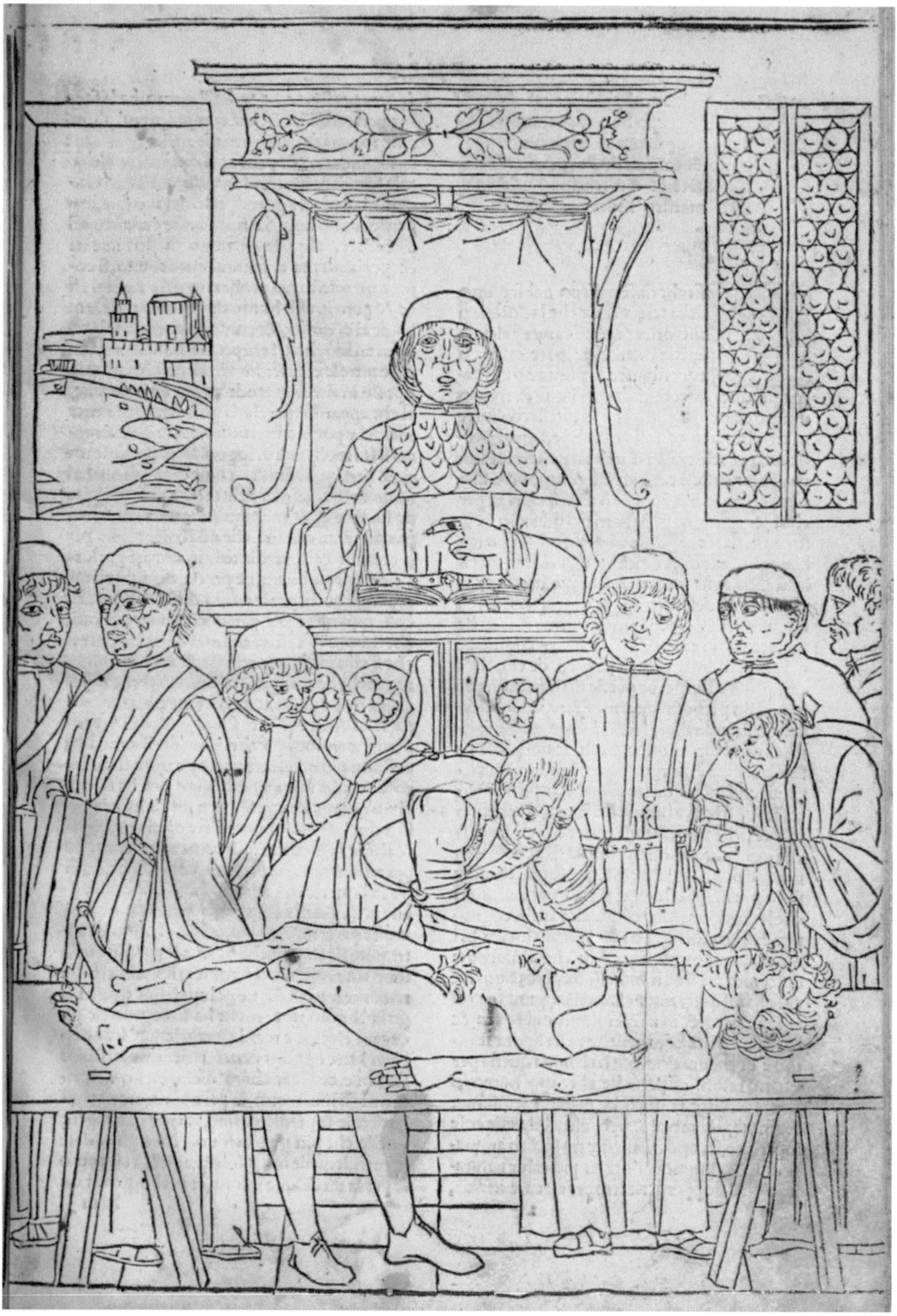

Fig. 1.1 Fifteenth-century Italian woodcut showing dissection/autopsy being performed, perhaps in the setting of a university. Note that the professor sits above the group reading to them from a standard text, most likely Galen. (Courtesy of the National Library of Medicine)

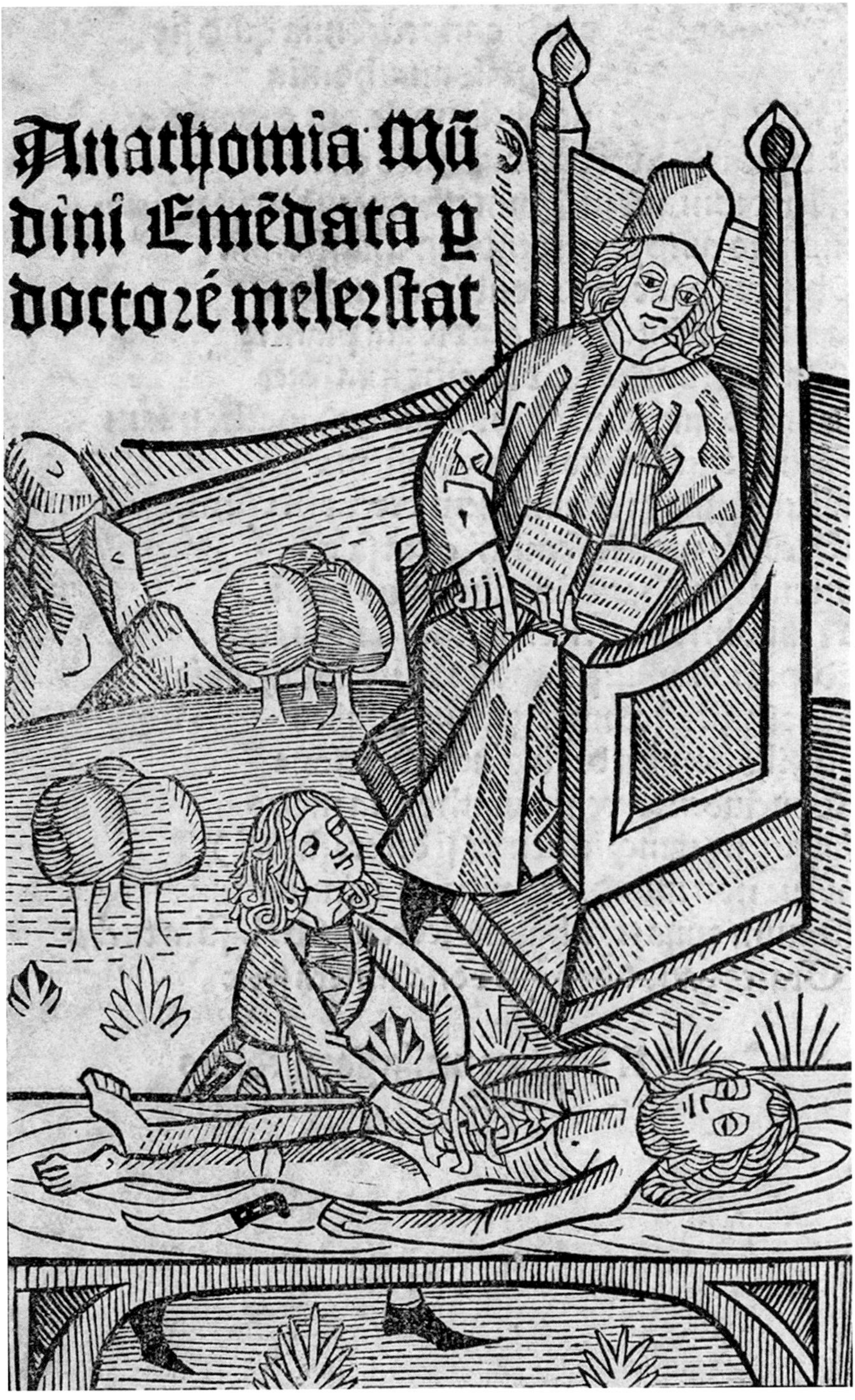

Fig. 1.2 Frontispiece of Mundinus' *Anathomia*. Note that Mundinus is not himself performing the dissection which is being carried out by an assistant, perhaps Alessandra Giliani. (Courtesy of the National Library of Medicine)

there is neither a definite time nor person that can be identified as having altered the focus of dissections from the discovery of anatomic structures to the revealing of the morphologic basis of disease, Benivieni and his work are an early example of that change.

The University of Padua became the great seat of learning for anatomy and pathology [22–25]. In 1341, **Gentile da Foligno** (1280–1348) carried out a public dissection at Padua. Subsequently the popularity of dissections increased. Soon after this public postmortem examinations were being carried out in Siena, in 1348, in Montpelier in 1366, Venice in 1368, Florence in 1388, and Paris in 1478, where dissections became a requirement for faculty members [1, 6]. At Padua, which accepted students from all nations and of all religions, the student body included **Nicolaus Copernicus** (1473–1543), who formulated the modern view of our universe (*De revolutionibus orbium coelestium*, published in 1543, the year of Copernicus' death and the year Vesalius published *De fabrica*); **William Harvey** (1578–1657), who went on to explain the circulation of the blood (*De motu cordis*, 1628) and also performed autopsies on many of his patients, including the ostensibly 152-year-old Thomas Parr in 1635; and **Galileo** (1564–1642), one of the greatest scientists of all time. Galileo went on to be a faculty member at Padua; his lecture platform is still preserved [23].

Legions of great physicians devoted themselves to discovering anatomic structures, including **Gabriele Falloppio** ("Fallopius") (1523–1562), one of the first to challenge the teachings of Galen, who described many of the structures of the female and male genital tracts; **Girolamo Fabrizio d'Acquapendente** ("Fabricius") (1533–1619), whose identification of the bursa that bears his name was vital in the development of modern immunology; **Giulio Cesare Aranzio** (Aranti) (1530–1589), who described the ductus arteriosus, the *corpora arantii* of the heart, and pioneered studies of the fetus; and **Bartolomeo Eustachio** (1500–1574), originally an ardent Galenist who became an enthusiastic Vesalian and who discovered the auditory tube that bears his name, the thoracic duct, and the adrenal glands. Others, at Padua and elsewhere, whose names are engraved in the lexicon of medicine, flourished in this era (e.g., **Marco degli Oddi** (1526–1591), who identified the duodenal sphincter of the common bile duct; **Adriaan van den Spiegel** ("Spigelius") (1578–1625), who wrote about the muscles and fasciae of the abdominal wall as well as the caudate lobe of the liver ("Spiegel lobe"); **Antonio Valsalva** (1666–1723), whose name is associated with the Valsalva maneuver, a test of circulatory function, and who made various anatomic contributions, as well as many others who practiced medicine and studied human structure [1, 6, 23, 26].

Andreas Vesalius Corrects Galen

It was **Andreas Vesalius** (1514–1564) who provided the first and most important step in establishing medicine as a scientific discipline [22–24]. His monumental *De humani corporis fabrica libri septem* ("the structure of the human body in seven books; *De fabrica*") corrected the many errors and misinterpretations of Galenic anatomy. It was illustrated in part by Vesalius himself but mostly by Stephen von Calcar, a student of Titian. In contrast to generally accepted practice reflected in many illustrations of the time, in which a teacher directed someone else, Vesalius performed the dissections himself. Vesalius came to Padua after being in Paris and Louvain. His epochal achievements overthrew the more than 1000 years of Galenic influence on medicine. **William Osler** (1849–1919) later described Vesalius' 1543 *De fabrica* as the greatest medical book ever written and the start of modern medicine (Fig. 1.3). In addition to the original Latin, *De fabrica* was published in German, allowing for its use in many countries. **Ambroise Paré** (1510–1590), the greatest Renaissance surgeon, read the translated version and immediately recognized the importance of *De fabrica*. Paré became a significant force in spreading Vesalius' teaching [1, 21].

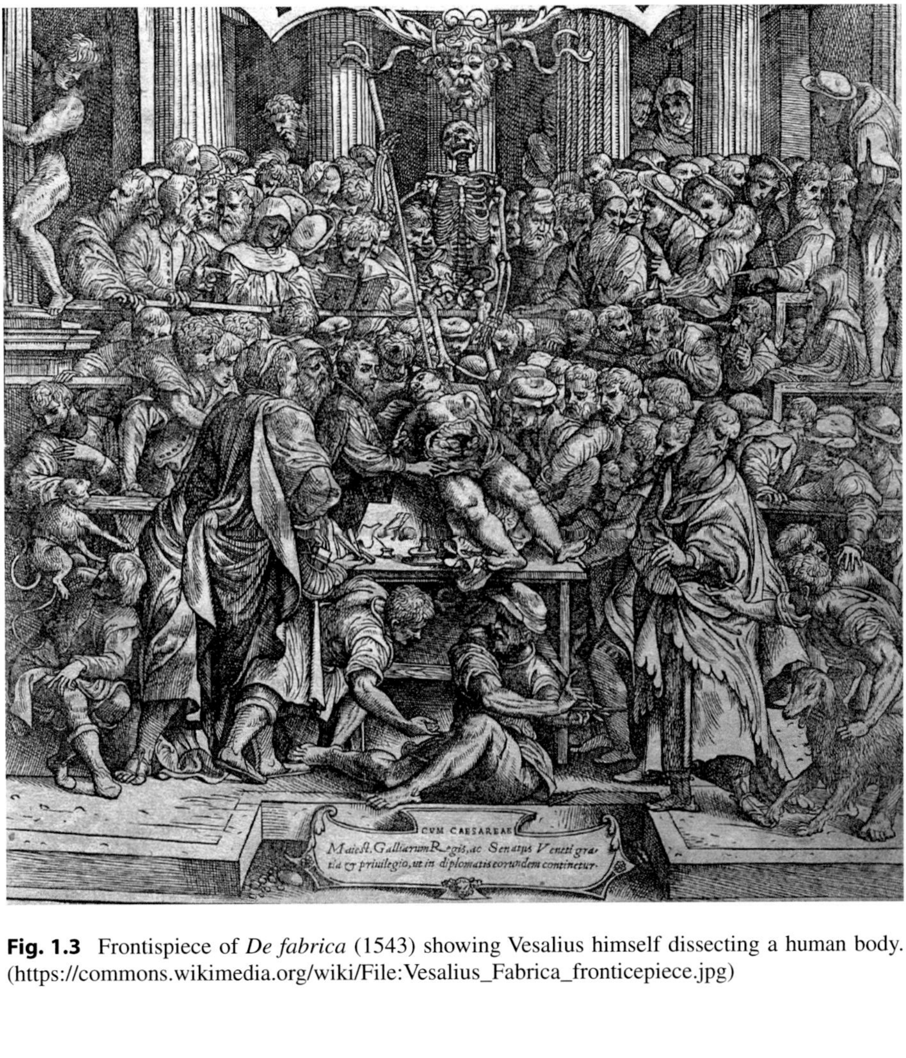

Fig. 1.3 Frontispiece of *De fabrica* (1543) showing Vesalius himself dissecting a human body. (https://commons.wikimedia.org/wiki/File:Vesalius_Fabrica_fronticepiece.jpg)

In the next four centuries, human dissections were increasingly employed in Europe and in the New World. Indeed, the first recorded human dissection in the western hemisphere was performed 10 years before the publication of *De fabrica* in what is now the Dominican Republic, on the bodies of conjoined twins [8].

The Coming of Age of The Autopsy

Morgagni Shows that Disease Is Founded in Morphologic Alterations

It remained for **Giovanni Battista Morgagni** (1682–1771) (Fig. 1.4), a student of Valsalva at Bologna before he came to Padua, to transform human dissections from anatomic exercises to a vital component of the medical care of the patient who has died. At the age of 79, in 1761, Morgagni recorded the observations of a lifetime in his great work *De sedibus et causis morborum per anatomen indagatis* (*De sedibus*) (the sites and causes of disease established by anatomic investigations) confirming once and for all the principle that human diseases are founded in morphologic alterations. A profound and tireless student of disease, given the chair of anatomy at Padua at the age of 33, Morgagni differed from his predecessors in applying logical reasoning to groups of cases, rather than only collecting isolated observations. Fully entitled to a preeminent position in the history of medicine for establishing postmortem examinations as the scientific basis of medical study to identify pathogenesis and the course of diseases, he was also one of the greatest contributors to clinical medical practice and diagnosis, describing a host of diseases and conditions, including cirrhosis, various tumors, brain abscess as a sequel to otitis media, hemiplegia as a sequel to contralateral brain injury, pneumonic "hepatization,"

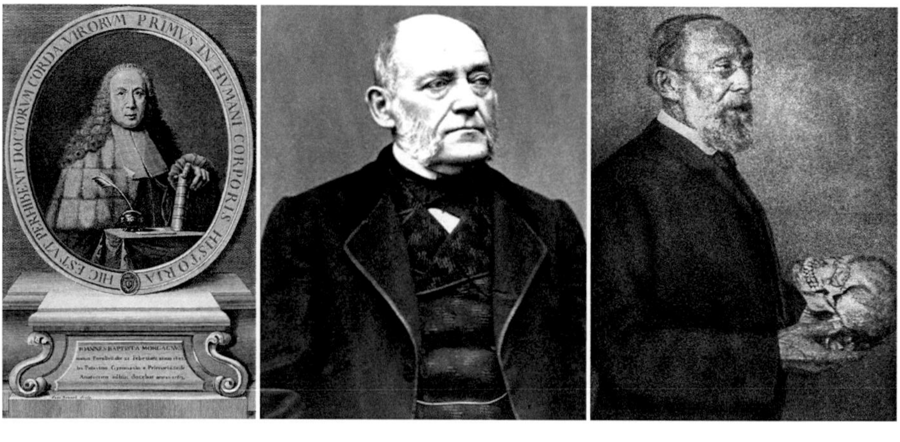

Fig. 1.4 Images of Giovanni Batista Morgagni, Karl von Rokitansky, and Rudolf Virchow. (https://commons.wikimedia.org/wiki/File:G._B._Morgagni,_%22De_sedibus...%22,_1761;_title_page_Wellcome_L0000576.jpg)

pulmonary tuberculosis, aortic syphilis, gummata of the liver and brain, vegetative endocarditis, aneurysm, tetralogy of Fallot, Stokes-Adams syndrome, Turner-Albright syndrome, gastric carcinoma, colonic carcinoma, probably Crohn's disease, and literally dozens of others, as well as many anatomic structures.

Modern medicine owes its development to Padua, with the foundations set by Vesalius, the anatomist, Harvey, the physiologist, and Morgagni, the pathologist [25].

The Nineteenth Century

In the early nineteenth century, building on the firm foundation established by Morgagni, great contributions to medical knowledge were made through autopsy by many physicians: **Herman Boerhaave** (1668–1738), regarded as the founder of clinical teaching and of the modern academic hospital; **Joseph Lieutaud** (1703–1780), who eventually became physician to Louis XVI of France; **Matthew Baillie** (1761–1823), author of the first English language pathology text; **Marie-Francois Xavier Bichat** (1771–1802), who demonstrated the variability of tissues and has been called "father of histology"; Bichat's student **René Theophile Hyacinthe Laennec** (1781–1826), a great pulmonary pathologist who invented the stethoscope; **P.C.A. Louis** (1787–1872), who brought statistical studies to medicine; and **Thomas Hodgkin** (1798–1865), a great educator and humanitarian who described the disease that bears his name and also delineated the features separating inflammation from neoplasia. Diseases were, for the first time, recognized, and their pathogenesis began to be understood. Hodgkin created one of the first pathology specimen museums (now known as the "Gordon Museum" at Guy's Hospital, London) organized by systems for student and physician education. He was an important proponent of the autopsy and one of the first physicians to devote himself almost entirely to autopsy performance [32]. Hodgkin might well be regarded as the first full-time pathologist, although that appellation could as well be applied to Erasistratus, Benivieni, Morgagni, or **Karl Rokitansky** (1804–1878).

Karl Rokitansky: Expanding on Morgagni

Karl Rokitansky, in Vienna in the mid-nineteenth century, performed more than 30,000 autopsies himself and examined another 60,000 (Fig. 1.4) [1, 2, 8–12, 33, 34]. Most importantly he was the first to study the pathologic changes he found at autopsy in a systematic manner, carefully correlating the morphologic observations with the clinical events. He expanded the Morgagni principle, permanently establishing the tradition of clinical-pathologic correlation and confirming the key role of the pathologist in the study of human disease. Founder of the great Viennese school of Pathology, Rokitansky was a brilliant observer with an extraordinary breadth and depth of experience. Despite this, Rokitansky inexplicably held to the primitive theory that diseases were due to either "crasias" or "dyscrasias." To his credit,

Rokitansky, perhaps the most renowned physician in the world in the mid-nineteenth century, publicly abandoned this outdated concept after learning the work and theories of **Rudolf Virchow** (1821–1902) in Berlin.

Rudolf Virchow and Cell Theory

Rudolf Virchow (Fig. 1.4), certainly one of the greatest figures in the history of pathology and of medicine, developed the seminal concept that disease begins in the cell and not with mysterious humors ("omnis cellula e cellula"; all cells (come) from cells) [35, 36]. A scientist, teacher, anthropologist, and social revolutionary, Virchow initiated the transformation of medicine from art to modern science, setting the stage for the development of surgical pathology and, in a sense, even molecular pathology, because of his insights about the origins of diseases. Although he was not the first to use the microscope in studying human tissues, his teachings were instrumental in altering the approach to the autopsy, which had been principally based on macroscopic observations. Virchow emphasized the need for standardization of procedures [37], in 1876. Four years previously, in 1872, **Francis Delafield** (1841–1915), at New York's College of Physicians and Surgeons, founder of the first pathology laboratory in the United States, published his autopsy text, emphasizing the same need [38].

The understanding of Virchow's cell theory opened the doors to the molecular studies of the twenty-first century, just as Vesalius, Harvey, and Morgagni opened the doors to the great diagnostic and therapeutic advances of the twentieth century [39].

The great medical thinkers over the past 2500 years and their contributions to the development of human dissection and to the autopsy are listed in Table 1.1.

Table 1.1 Key figures in the history of human dissection and of the autopsy

Key figure	Time period	Country/Region	Major contribution
Herophilus	335–280 BCE	Greece	First person to search into causes of disease through human dissection
Galen	138–201	Rome	Detailed descriptions of anatomic structures; first to demonstrate arterial pulsations, function of laryngeal nerve, ureters, and many other aspects of anatomy
Vesalius	1514–1564	Padua/Paris/Louvain	Established medicine as a scientific discipline and corrected the many errors and misinterpretations of Galenic anatomy
Morgagni	1682–1771	Padua/Bologna	Confirmed once and for all the principle that human diseases are founded in morphologic alterations
Rokitansky	1804–1878	Vienna	Expanded on the Morgagni principle by correlating morphologic observations with clinical events and confirmed the role of the pathologist in the study of human disease
Virchow	1821–1902	Germany	Developed the seminal concept that disease begins in the cell rather than with mysterious humors and transformed medicine from art to modern science

The Twentieth Century

The twentieth century saw the greatest expansion in the use of the autopsy worldwide, reaching its peak of development in Vienna and Berlin before World War I and in the United States in the years before and after World War II. A list of the disorders understood in the twentieth century on the basis of autopsy includes influenza, systemic lupus erythematosus and other collagen-vascular diseases, rheumatic fever, Legionnaire's disease, the nature and behavior of most tumors including brain tumors, and acquired immunodeficiency syndrome (AIDS), to name just a few. The many autopsies performed, and their recording in the medical literature, greatly advanced medical knowledge and scientific investigation, improved the quality of medical care, and benefited society in terms of forensics and environmental control. The autopsy improved understanding of the efficacy and deleterious effects of therapies, including radiation and chemotherapy. Information provided to family members about possible genetic and infectious implications proved invaluable to them and, as studies have shown, also helped to relieve guilt, lessen the pain of grieving, and shorten the mourning period.

By the end of the twentieth century, the numbers of autopsies performed throughout the world declined, despite the continuing documentation of its usefulness and also despite the fact that as many as 15–40% of patients still die without an established correct clinical diagnosis, even when the most sophisticated techniques have been applied [40–45]. The 1983 hallmark article by Goldman and co-workers about discrepancies between the most significant clinical diagnoses and the most significant autopsy findings showed that "advances in diagnostic technology have not reduced the value of the autopsy" [46]. This conclusion has, more than three decades later, been again confirmed: "despite intensive modern clinical investigations, autopsies continue to reveal major antemortem diagnostic errors in a significant number of cases" [47]. It is not possible to calculate the enormous amount of information about human disorders, particularly, about the pathogenesis of disorders, that has been lost in recent years because of the failure to perform autopsies in more than 95% of people who die in hospitals. Many reasons can be cited for this troubling decline, including economic factors, decline of emphasis of autopsy in medical schools, fear of litigation among clinicians, misplaced confidence in the degree of reliability of modern diagnostic methods, and lack of complete understanding about social and religious customs that may affect the autopsy [48–55].

Observations on The Future of The Autopsy

With renewed and increasing recognition of the continuing value of a thoughtfully performed and reported autopsy, efforts are being made to restore the autopsy to an appropriate level of utilization for the benefit of humankind.

As the sciences of molecular medicine and molecular pathology become increasingly sophisticated and specific, there may be a time when diagnostic markers for every known condition are determined and all currently known diagnostic approaches, both invasive and noninvasive, become unnecessary. It is no longer beyond the realm of imagination to expect that a tiny sample of blood or other biologic material could be studied to reveal all abnormalities in the body. It is even conceivable that some handheld scanning device similar to that used by Dr. Leonard McCoy ("Bones") in the science fiction series *Star Trek* will be available. When that time will be is impossible to determine, but it is highly unlikely to occur in the next 20 years. Until that time, and probably longer than that, the autopsy remains an invaluable component of medical care as study after study demonstrates significant diagnostic discrepancy rates of 10–25% even in the best-equipped medical centers [47, 56, 57].

Unfortunately, it may well be that the well-performed, "complete" hospital autopsy will cease to exist in the coming decade, even in academic centers, because of a combination of clinician and pathologist disinterest, lack of effectiveness of individual pathologists and their organizations in explaining to both the medical profession and lay public the continuing benefits of autopsy, and economic factors such as health insurers not paying for autopsy and hospital administrators not supporting autopsy. Although many currently practicing pathologists understand well the high value of the autopsy and are skilled in its performance [58–60], increasing numbers of young pathologists may not be capable of performing complete autopsies [61]. New pathologists, at the beginning of their careers, typically have performed only the minimum required number of autopsies when they complete their residency. There are examples throughout the country where hospital autopsies are performed by forensic pathologists who, though highly qualified to investigate death, may not approach the hospital autopsy in the traditional way. For many years, there has been the suggestion that regional autopsy centers be established to allow for autopsy performance by committed and experienced pathologists and some centers currently exist [62].

Suggestions for improving and reviving the autopsy have been made in recent years [58, 63] and employing these and other new ideas can further add to the autopsy's value. However, efforts to "modernize" the autopsy will still require considerable effort on the economic and political fronts to ensure that the autopsy continues to serve the medical profession and the public at large.

References

1. Castiglioni A. A history of medicine. 2nd ed. New York: Alfred A. Knopf; 1947.
2. Mettler CC. History of medicine. Philadelphia: Blakiston; 1947.
3. Singer CJ. A short history of anatomy from the Greeks to Harvey. New York: Dover Publications; 1957.
4. Kevorkian J. The story of dissection. New York: Philosophical Library; 1959.
5. Spiro RK. A backward glance at the study of postmortem anatomy. Part 1. Int Surg. 1971;56:27–40.
6. Spiro RK. A backward glance at the study of postmortem anatomy. Part 2. Int Surg. 1971;56:101–12.
7. Stenn F. Six hundred years of autopsies. Lab Med. 1971;2:21–5.
8. King LS, Meehan MC. A history of the autopsy. Am J Path. 1973;73:514–44.

9. Porter R. The greatest benefit to mankind. New York: W.W. Norton; 1998.
10. Burton JL, Rutty G. The history of the autopsy. In: Burton JL, Rutty G, editors. The hospital autopsy. London: Hodder Arnold; 2010. p. 1–10.
11. Connolly AJ, Finkbeiner WE, Ursell PC, Davis RL. The autopsy – past and present. In: Connolly AJ, Finkbeiner WE, Ursell PC, Davis RL, editors. Autopsy pathology: a manual and atlas. 3rd ed. Philadelphia: Elsevier; 2017.
12. Geller SA. A short history of the autopsy. In: Hutchins GM, Collins K, editors. Autopsy performance and reporting. 2nd ed. IL, College of American Pathologists: Northfield; 2003. p. 1–9.
13. van den Tweel JG, Taylor CR. The age of the autopsy. In: van den Tweel JG, Gu J, Taylor CR, editors. From magic to molecules – an illustrated history of disease. Beijing: Peking University Press; 2016. p. 65–80.
14. Skinner HA. The origin of medical terms. New York: Hafner; 1970. p. 54.
15. MoyerE.DustingoffaTreasure:cleaningandrehousingtheLaddcollection.https://nyamcenterforhistory.org/2014/10/01/dusting-off-a-treasures-cleaning-and-rehousing-the-ladd-collection/.
16. Gordon BL. Medicine among the ancient Hebrews. Ann Med Hist, Series III. 1935;2:219–35.
17. Goodman NR, Goodman JL, Hofman WI. Autopsy: traditional Jewish laws and customs "Halacha". Am J Forensic Med Pathol. 2011;32:300–3.
18. Rosner F. Julius Preuss' biblical and talmudic medicine. New York: Hebrew Publishing Company; 1978.
19. Persaud TVN. Early history of human anatomy: from antiquity to the beginning of the modern era. Charles C. Thomas: Springfield; 1984.
20. Bay NS, Bay BH. Greek anatomist Herophilus: the father of anatomy. Anat Cell Bioly. 2010;43:280–3.
21. Gross CG. Galen and the squealing pig. Neurosci. 1998;4:216–21.
22. O'Malley CD. Andreas Vesalius of Brussels, 1514–1564. Berkeley: University of California Press; 1964.
23. Rossetti L. The University of Padua. Edizioni Lint: Trieste; 1983.
24. Geller SA. Il Bo – the foundations of modern medicine are established. In: Thiene G, Pessina AC, editors. Advances in cardiovascular medicine. Padova: Univ Degli Studi di Padova; 2002. p. 309–36.
25. Geller SA. Renaissance anatomists. In: van Tweel JG, Gu J, Taylor CR, editors. From magic to molecules – an illustrated history of disease. Beijing: Peking University Medical Press; 2016. p. 49–64.
26. Proskauer C. The significance to medical history of the newly discovered fourth century roman fresco. Bull NY Acad Med. 1958;34:672–86.
27. Wolf-Heidiger G, Cetto M. Anatomical dissection in pictorial representation. Ciba Symp. 1957;5:124–6, 168–72.
28. Wolf-Heidiger G, Cetto AM. Die anatomische Sektion in bildlicher Darstellung. Basel: Verlag S Karger; 1967. p. 36.
29. Medici M. Compendio storico della Scuola anatomica di Bologna; 1857. p. 28–30. (https://books.google.com/books?id+HZqnnF0hwd8C&pg+PA29).
30. Giliani A. https:\\en.wikipedia.org/wik/Alessandra_Giliani.
31. Quick B. A Golden Web. New York: HarperTeen; 2010.
32. Geller SA, Taylor C. Thomas Hodgkin, the "man" and the "disease": humani nihil se alienum putabit (nothing human was foreign to him). Virchows Arch. 2013;463:353–85.
33. King LS. The medical world of the eighteenth century. Huntington: Robert E. Krieger Publishing; 1958.
34. Lesky E. The Vienna medical school of the 19th century. Baltimore: Johns Hopkins University Press; 1976.
35. Ackernecht EH. Rudolf Virchow – doctor, statesman, anthropologist. Madison, University of Wisconsin Press; 1953.
36. Virchow R. Die Cellularpathologie. Berlin: August Hirschwald; 1858, (original American version: Virchow R. Cellular Pathology. Tr. by Frank Chance, Philadelphia, J.B. Lippincott and Co., 1863).

37. Virchow R. Die Sektions Technik im Leinchenhause des Charité-Krankenhauses. 3rd ed. Berlin: August Hirshwald; 1884, (original American version: Virchow R. Post-mortem Examinations. Tr. by Smith TP. Philadelphia, Lindsay & Blakiston, 1877).
38. Delafield FA. Handbook of postmortem examination and morbid anatomy, 1872.
39. McCusick VA. The anatomy of the human genome: a neo-Vesalian basis for medicine in the 21st century. JAMA. 2001;286:2289–95.
40. Geller SA. To see or not to see; the status of the autopsy at the Mount Sinai Medical Center. Mt Sinai J Med. 1979;46:33–8.
41. McPhee SJ, Bottles K. Autopsy: moribund art or vital science. Am J Med. 1985;78:107–13.
42. Sinard JH. Factors affecting autopsy rates, autopsy request rates, and autopsy findings at a large academic medical center. Exp Mol Pathol. 2001;70:333–43.
43. Burton EC, Phillips RS, Covinsky KE, et al. The relation of autopsy rate to physicians' beliefs and recommendations regarding autopsy. Am J Med. 2004;117:255–61.
44. Ayoub T, Chow J. The conventional autopsy in modern medicine. J R Soc Med. 2008;101:177–81.
45. Turnbull A, Osborn M, Nicholas N. Hospital autopsy: endangered or extinct? J Clin Pathol. 2015;68:601–4.
46. Goldman L, Sayson R, Robbins S, et al. The value of the autopsy in three medical eras. N Engl J Med. 1983;308:1000–5.
47. Marshall HS, Milikowski C. Comparison of clinical diagnoses and autopsy findings. Arch Pathol Lab Med. 2017;141:1262–6.
48. Forbes TR. Crowner's quest. Trans Am Philosophical Soc. 1978;68:1–52.
49. Ball JM. The body snatchers. New York: Dorset Press; 1989.
50. Geller SA. Religious attitudes and the autopsy. Arch Pathol Lab Med. 1984;108:494–6.
51. Davis GJ, Patterson BR. Dilemmas and solutions of the pathologists and clinician encountering religious views of the autopsy. South Med J. 1996;89:1041–4.
52. Chakraborty R, El-Jawahri AR, Litzow MR, et al. A systematic review of religious beliefs about major end-of-life issues in the five major world religions. Palliat Support Care. 2017;15:609–22.
53. Mohammed M, Kharoshah MA. Autopsy in Islam and current practice in Arab Muslim countries. J Forensic Legal Med. 2014;23:80–3.
54. Sajid MI. Autopsy in Islam: considerations for deceased Muslims and their families currently and in the future. Am J Forensic Med Pathol. 2016;37:29–31.
55. Hooper J, Geller SA. Relevance of the autopsy as a medical tool: a large database of physician attitudes. Arch Pathol Lab Med. 2007;131:268–74.
56. Winters B, Custer J, Galvagno SM Jr, et al. Diagnostic errors in the intensive care unit: a systematic review of autopsy studies. BMI Qual Saf. 2012;21:894–902.
57. McGuire AL, Moore Q, Majumber M, et al. The ethics of conducting molecular autopsies in cases of sudden death in the young. Genome Res. 2016;26:1165–9.
58. Goldman BI. Reviving the hospital autopsy. Arch Pathol Lab Med. 2016;140:503–4.
59. Krywanczyk A, Mount S. In defense of the academic autopsy. Arch Pathol Lab Med. 2018;142:157–8.
60. Wolf DW. A new kind of autopsy for 21st century medicine. Arch Pathol Lab Med. 2018;142:158.
61. Geller SA. Who will do my autopsy? Arch Pathol Lab Med. 2015;139:578–80.
62. Trelstad RL, Amenta PS, Foran DJ, Smilow PC. The role for regional autopsy centers in the evaluation of covered deaths. Survey of opinions of US and Canadian chairs of pathology and major health insurers in the United States. Arch Pathol Lab Med. 1996;120:753–8.
63. Laposata M. A new kind of autopsy for 21st century medicine. Arch Pathol Lab Med. 2017;141:887–8.

Part II

Demonstrating Value in Autopsy Practice

Utilizing the Autopsy for Quality Improvement

2

Harold Sanchez and Gregory Chamberlin

Introduction

Quality management (QM) as a distinct profession has its origins in industry, particularly manufacturing, in the early 1900s. Since then quality management techniques have been applied to almost every field of human endeavor, including medicine. Medical quality management (MQM) has become its own subspecialty with several professional societies, each with its own certification program, peer-reviewed journal, and annual meeting. The first section of this chapter will provide a basic introduction to QM history, terminology, and concepts. Several historical vignettes will be provided to illustrate a few relevant key concepts. Perhaps the most crucial concept to bear in mind for our purposes is that rational quality management is impossible without measurement.

QM is part of the everyday life of most laboratory professionals who are accustomed to assuring that freezers are cold, controls are within range, new procedures are validated, frozen section diagnoses correlate with final diagnoses, and lab staff is proficient. Meticulous records are kept and held ready for inspectors from a variety of oversight organizations. These familiar activities, which ensure the integrity of the process and quality of results, fall under the general heading of quality assurance (QA). Quality improvement (QI) is a cyclical, ongoing process.

It involves continuously evaluating policies and procedures, devising ways to improve them, implementing the proposed changes, and evaluating their effects. Intradepartmental QI projects are also part of the ongoing work of the laboratory. Autopsy data can also be used as part of hospital-wide QI initiatives. The second section of this chapter will discuss autopsy QA and the use of autopsy as part of institutional QI.

H. Sanchez (✉) · G. Chamberlin
Frank H. Netter MD School of Medicine at Quinnipiac University, North Haven, CT, USA
e-mail: harold.sanchez@yale.edu; gregory.chamberlin@quinnipiac.edu

J. E. Hooper, A. K. Williamson (eds.), *Autopsy in the 21st Century*,
https://doi.org/10.1007/978-3-319-98373-8_2

Finally, autopsy results have the proven potential to impact patient outcomes when applied to QI projects beyond an individual hospital. This last application of autopsy results is the most challenging and potentially the most important. Recent years have seen an increased national interest in improving patient care by reducing medical errors and improving the diagnostic process. The third section of this chapter will discuss the role that the autopsy can play in a broad national effort to improve patient outcomes. The autopsy is an indispensable tool for obtaining the measurements needed to monitor and ultimately improve the clinical diagnostic process.

Quality Management

Quality management was created to further the financial interests of its practitioners. It evolved under the selective pressure of industrial and military competition. New management approaches both succeeded and proliferated because they yielded financial success or failed because they did not. Even the emphasis on the customer (or in the case of medicine, the patient) can be viewed, in part, through a business lens. In short, QM is not window dressing. QM is an essential ingredient in the success of any large organization that operates in a competitive environment, and QM is not possible without measurement. A brief review of the history of the field will serve to illustrate this (more comprehensive reviews can be found in the reference section) [1–4].

Quality Management History

Medieval trade guilds were influential commercial organizations that strove to create local monopolies on their goods and services. One key ingredient in that effort was the reliably high quality of their products. The guilds maintained high standards for raw materials (with thorough inspections and severe penalties for shoddy suppliers) and workmanship (through a detailed apprenticeship program). Master craftsmen inspected the finished goods and only affixed their seal of approval to those that met their standards. This was not just a matter of professional or civic pride. The quality of the finished product ensured their reputation, and their reputation assured their livelihood.

The dramatic technical advances of the Industrial Revolution changed the speed and scale of production. Factories consumed raw materials in quantities too large to be completely inspected. Finished goods were produced at high speed in large volumes, and mistakes in the production process became very expensive to address. Qualitative standards were no longer adequate. The entire manufacturing process was subjected to minute quantitative analysis. Measurements were taken and benchmarks and standards were created.

This approach created a demand for trained managers and efficiency specialists. Frederick W. Taylor's *Principles of Scientific Management* (published in 1911) was the start of industrial engineering and made Taylor the first management consultant.

The cost of QM and efficiency experts was more than offset by the savings in waste and the improvement in the quality of the finished product.

The success of Taylor's approach to eliminating waste and inefficiency generated interest in applying similar techniques to other sectors of society. Reforms in medical education (e.g., the *Flexner Report*) and hospital administration were heavily influenced by the movement [5].

In the 1920s, Western Electric engineer Walter Shewhart revolutionized the approach to QM by developing the concept of statistical process control and introducing control charts. Shewhart followers like W. Edwards Deming would promote and expand on his work. The power of the statistical approach to QM was demonstrated in the US manufacturing effort in World War II and in the miraculous rise of Japanese manufacturing in the 1950s, 1960s, and 1970s.

Modern Quality Management

The late 1960s also saw the beginnings of medical quality management (MQM) as a separate discipline [6] driven in part by the demands of sprawling new federal programs like Medicare and Medicaid. Physician researchers analyzed health-care delivery as a system, identified opportunities for improvement, and proposed measures (performance monitoring, peer review, improvements in medical and professional education) to address deficiencies. Among the earliest influential work was that of Avedis Donabedian [7].

In the 1980s Motorola developed a program called Six Sigma to dramatically decrease product defects and improve customer satisfaction. The goal was to reduce defects to 3.4 defects per million opportunities (3.4 DPMO) through QI projects that were data driven, time bound, and supported by management. Central to the success of these QI projects was the application of a process, DMAIC: define, measure, analyze, improve, and control. Simplistically, the target defect and expected improvements are defined, validated data is measured to establish a baseline, the data is analyzed to identify vital few root causes of defects, a program is designed to improve the outcomes, and when improvements are achieved, the process is controlled to lock in gains. The initial investment in training and planning was documented to be more than offset over several years by substantial savings in production costs, improvements in customer satisfaction, and increases in profit. This approach has been adopted beyond the manufacturing industry and has been increasingly applied to hospital administration and health care.

Quality Management Vignettes

A well-designed, thoroughly integrated QM program provides an organization with tangible benefits and more than justifies the associated costs. A poorly designed, halfheartedly applied program can be disastrous. In this subsection, several examples (medical and otherwise) of successful and unsuccessful applications of management principles are offered to illustrate several important points that will be applied later to a consideration of the use of autopsy data in QM.

Vignette #1: The Ford Pinto

In the 1970s the Ford Motor Company responded to a flood of fuel-efficient compact imports by designing the Pinto. Product development was proceeding at record-setting pace until crash tests revealed potentially dangerous design flaws in the rear-mounted gas tank. Against the advice of engineers, Ford decided to continue with production and to absorb the costs of litigation resulting from any injuries and deaths. What followed was a horrendous toll in human suffering, enormous civil lawsuits, and the first criminal charges ever brought against an American company for faulty product design [8].

Lessons: *Emphasizing speed and short-term profits over the interests of the customer (or patient), in addition to being unconscionable, is ultimately bad for the organization. The cost and inconvenience of instituting and sticking to a sound QM program are ultimately much less than the cost of not having one or circumventing one.*

Vignette #2: Commercial Cytology Laboratories

The 1970s and 1980s saw the advent of large commercial cytology laboratories which were able to offer lower costs than hospital labs because of larger volumes and an inexpensive workforce. Cytotechnologists were paid on a piecework basis in a system that incentivized speed and volume. Professional societies expressed their alarm, but commercial laboratories countered that they had quality assurance measures in place, complied with state statutes, and passed state inspections.

Print and television journalism [9] exposed the harsh working conditions and highlighted missed diagnoses that led to tragic outcomes. The federal government responded with the Clinical Laboratory Improvement Amendments (CLIA) in 1988 and a program of mandatory annual proficiency testing for all pathologists who reviewed Pap smears. The Pap smear remains the only anatomic specimen type that is subjected to targeted proficiency testing. There is no data to indicate that the testing has led to improved diagnoses.

Lessons: *Simply having a nominal QM program does not ensure quality results. Failure to regulate the quality of medical care from within the system can lead to well-meaning but ineffective (and onerous) external regulation.*

Vignette #3: Ignaz Semmelweis and Ernest Codman [10]

In the 1840s, Ignaz Semmelweis published his work showing that handwashing dramatically lowered the rate of postpartum sepsis and maternal mortality at a prestigious Vienna hospital [11, 12]. The European obstetric community was unconvinced despite Semmelweis' impassioned (and later vitriolic) advocacy supported by what seemed like irrefutable evidence. Semmelweis died in obscurity in an asylum at the age of 47.

Born 4 years after Semmelweis' death, Ernest Amory Codman was a respected Boston orthopedic surgeon at the Massachusetts General Hospital. He developed an ambitious QI program which involved following up on all of his patients after discharge to assess the accuracy of diagnosis and the effectiveness of therapy. He urged hospitals to follow his example and use the resulting data to monitor quality and make decisions about promotions. He was largely ignored. Nevertheless, he advocated zealously (and stridently) for his program [13]. As a result he lost his position at the hospital, his professional standing suffered, and he ended life buried in an unmarked grave.

Lessons: *Neither the weight of evidence, nor expert opinion, nor zealous individual advocacy is sufficient to change entrenched opinions and challenge vested interests.*

Vignette #4: The Tissue Committee

Part of the response to the shortage of hospital beds in the 1940s and 1950s was utilization review. Reviews of medical records and pathology reports had made it clear that certain low-risk surgical procedures (hysterectomies, oophorectomies, appendectomies, tonsillectomies) were often performed without compelling indications and produced surgical specimens that were free of discernible pathology.

Tissue committees provided an extremely effective solution. Typically composed of surgeons, pathologists, and administrators, the committee reviewed preoperative records, operative notes, and pathology reports and made determinations on the appropriateness of a procedure. Statistics were compiled for individual surgeons and for the hospital. When needed, focused corrective plans were devised.

Tissue committees were a very cost-effective means of reducing the rates of unnecessary procedures. Some of the first influential literature reports on tissue committees came from small community hospitals [14–16].

Lessons: *Medical quality management can produce significant improvements in patient outcomes. This can be accomplished in hospitals of any size with modest investments of staff time and hospital funds. Active participation of stakeholders across clinical departments and the administration is crucial. Pathologists can (and should) play a central role.*

Autopsy Quality Assurance and Quality Improvement

With the historical underpinnings and general principles of quality management discussed in the previous section of the chapter, this section serves to outline the practical considerations for assuring the quality of a medical institution's autopsy service.

As mentioned earlier, the federal government enacted the Clinical Laboratory Improvement Amendments of 1988 (CLIA) to regulate all laboratory testing (with the exception of research) performed on humans in the USA. Presently the Centers for Medicare & Medicaid Services (CMS) oversees the implementation of CLIA. Laboratories can be directly inspected by CMS to attain a Certificate of Compliance with CLIA. However, the CMS also offers a Certificate of Accreditation to laboratories that are accredited with a CMS-approved accreditation organization. The College of American Pathologists (CAP) is one such organization. The CAP represents the largest organization of pathologists certified by the American Board of Pathology and is considered a world leader in laboratory accreditation and proficiency testing. As such, many laboratories associated with hospitals have chosen to become CAP accredited in order to show compliance with CLIA.

CAP Accreditation

The CAP's accreditation program is carried out through the use of several checklists which are updated yearly to reflect advancements in laboratory medicine. The CAP includes regulations regarding the practice of autopsy within its Anatomic Pathology Checklist. Given the substantial number of laboratories adhering to the CAP accreditation standards to achieve CLIA compliance (as well as the comprehensive nature of the CAP's attention to autopsy), this section will heavily reference the CAP checklist when discussing best practices for autopsy. Please note that, at the time of writing, the most current CAP checklist was released in August 2017 and a more updated version may now be available.

Figure 2.1 is a visual representation of the current CAP accreditation standards for autopsy proceedings. The checklist items most vital to maintaining a suitable work environment provide the foundation for the autopsy quality assurance pyramid. Each element of the pyramid is dependent on all the elements that lie below it in order to be incorporated into a successful autopsy service.

CAP arranges its checklist items according to "phase." The phase designation reflects the dangers posed if an institution is deficient in that checklist item. The phase also outlines how an institution must remediate should it be found to be deficient during an inspection. Phase 1 items do not have much of an effect on quality of care, and lack of compliance does not endanger the safety of personnel. Deficiencies in Phase 1 items require laboratories not only to correct the issue but also submit a written response to CAP outlining the changes made. No supportive documentation is required to back up said claims of remediation. Phase 2 items could have potentially significant impacts to both patient care and the well-being of staff. As such, institutions found to be deficient in Phase 2 items must submit an action plan to CAP as well as provide documentation to support the implementation of the proposed changes.

The CAP standards are clearly articulated, but what actually constitutes adequate evidence of compliance is left open to interpretation. Oftentimes "representative" autopsy cases will be chosen to highlight compliance with case-specific checklist

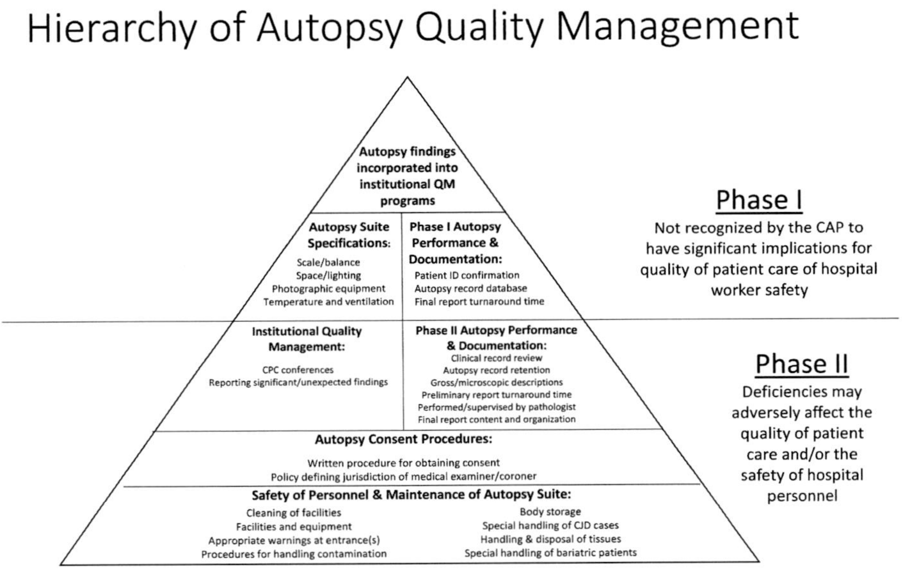

Fig. 2.1 Autopsy quality management evaluation pyramid

items, such as preliminary and final autopsy report turnaround times. However, this method may introduce significant bias as the few cases examined may not accurately reflect the service's performance as a whole.

It is the authors' opinion that documentation of compliance should be as thorough as possible, not only for the purposes of maintaining accreditation during inspections but to allow individual institutions to be able to apply the documentation toward quality improvement of the autopsy service itself. In this vein, we have included a series of logs and checklists at the end of this chapter that can be downloaded along with instructions for their intended uses. They can easily be incorporated into virtually any autopsy service's QA program. They serve as both comprehensive documentation of compliance and a means for an institution to quickly and accurately document improvement on deficient checklist items.

Autopsy Quality Specifications

First and foremost, the safety of the autopsy suite must be maintained. The entrance(s) to the autopsy suite must display signs warning of potential exposures to hazardous materials along with the need for universal precautions. The suite must also include appropriate personal protective equipment to protect skin and mucosal surfaces from both direct and aerosolized exposures. This equipment should either (1) be reusable with procedures in place for proper cleaning or (2) be single use with a method for disposal. Autopsy staff must have readily available and appropriate containers for contaminated waste and hazardous chemicals as well as written policies for their disposal present within the suite. The suite must contain written procedures for daily cleaning, cleaning following each autopsy, disposal of tissues, and handling of highly infectious cases. Written procedures are also required for cases where the patient's weight may pose an occupational hazard to autopsy staff. Finally, written procedures must also be present describing the proper handling of cases where prion diseases such as Creutzfeldt-Jakob disease are suspected. In order to properly store bodies, institutions must also have adequate refrigeration capabilities (with temperature logs showing temperatures maintained between 34 and 40 °F or between 1.1 and 4.4 °C) or embalming procedures.

Although designated as Phase 1, CAP outlines other requirements for the autopsy suite's physical layout and contents. The space available within the suite should be large enough to accommodate the average workload of the service, and the suite should be dedicated solely to the practice of autopsy and related endeavors (such as storage of tissues, teaching, etc.).

The space should also remain clean, maintain a comfortable ambient temperature, have adequate lighting, and provide adequate ventilation to control for airborne infectious agents. The suite should contain scales and/or balances that are calibrated periodically and that are appropriate for the types of cases performed in the suite (e.g., adult or fetal autopsy). Lastly the suite must have readily available photographic equipment to accurately document gross anatomy and pathology.

Autopsy Consent Procedures

Once safety of autopsy staff is assured, one must consider the consent procedure in place for requesting autopsy cases. The information that should be included in the consent document is a matter of much debate, and significant heterogeneity exists regarding when and how to approach next of kin for autopsy consent. Regardless of the method chosen, the minimum standards set forth by CAP require a written procedure for obtaining consent that details who may give consent. The order of precedence as to who is considered next of kin is subject to state statutes and thus may differ slightly from one institution to another. CAP standards also require clear guidelines for medical examiner or coroner jurisdiction and the assessment of whether a case should be treated as a medical or forensic autopsy. This will also be largely determined by state and local statutes or regulations.

Autopsy Performance

With appropriate safety and consent measures well-established, one can now consider the method in which the autopsy itself is conducted and the process of submitting reports detailing the autopsy findings.

A thorough autopsy must always begin with a review of the decedent's clinical records when available. Accurate and reliable information about the patient in life will direct both the questions that the autopsy can be expected to answer and the safety precautions that should be taken. Indeed, ignorance of the medical record can leave staff susceptible to exposure to any number of infectious agents, foreign bodies, hazardous chemicals, or sources of radioactivity [17]. The exact mechanism for obtaining the decedent's medical history can vary depending on what is available. Review of electronic health records or paper charts will often be the quickest method for obtaining necessary information. However, when possible, one should also "sign out" the case with a clinician who was directly involved in the care of the patient up to the point of death. Discussing the clinical course with an attending, fellow, or resident physician can offer a more comprehensive view of the decedent's health issues as well as open a dialogue between pathologist and clinician. Establishing such a line of communication has profound implications for the autopsy service. It targets the autopsy toward answering specific clinical questions and streamlines the reporting of findings to a clinician who knows to expect them.

Once the clinical history is well-understood, the autopsy practitioner should positively identify the body to be examined. Verification of the deceased should be confirmed using at least two independent identifiers prior to the first incision. A written procedure for identity verification must also be in place. The autopsy must either be performed or directly supervised by a pathologist who is certified by the American Board of Pathology in anatomic pathology (or who possesses equivalent qualifications).

Autopsy Documentation

A written preliminary anatomic diagnosis (PAD) should accompany the gross examination of the body. This report must be available to the attending clinician in charge of the decedent's care at the time of death within a reasonable timeframe. The expected turnaround time will vary depending on the extent of the autopsy. The CAP recommends a turnaround time of two working days for the majority of preliminary reports relying on gross examination only. This recommended timeframe is extended to four working days if the dissection is particularly complicated or if the PAD requires rush histology. If the case is limited to a single organ or a slide consultation, the preliminary report may be waived.

The final report must then be produced within 60 working days for 90% of cases. This timeline may be extended in particularly complex cases, especially when the need for outside consultation arises. However, if the final report does indeed require more than 60 days to complete, then the reason should be recorded, and the autopsy service director must document continued review of such cases. The content of the final report ought to be sufficiently comprehensive and well-organized such that a clinician can interpret the major disease processes present and identify the likely cause of death. Gross descriptions must be clear with detailed descriptions of any pathology identified. Assuming that microscopy is performed, the microscopic descriptions must be present in the final report. A key must also be included that details the blocks or slides from which the described microscopic findings are derived. The preliminary and final reports should be organized into a readily available database that allows for retrieval of cases by diagnosis. The specific type of database (electronic or otherwise) used can be chosen by the institution depending on its needs.

The retention of autopsy records represents the last consideration in this section. The CAP outlines its own required retention periods, which vary from one record type to another. Federal, state, and local laws may demand more or less stringent timeframes. Laboratories should maintain updated records of these laws and implement written policies that abide by whichever is the longest retention time for each record type.

Institutional Quality Management

The final aspect of the autopsy service to examine from a QA perspective is the use of autopsy results in the quality management efforts of the hospital at large. This involves not only the dissemination of information gleaned from autopsy to all relevant interested parties but also the multitude of ways in which this information can be used to improve the care of living patients.

As mentioned earlier, establishing a line of communication between autopsy staff and the clinicians who were treating the patient at the time of death can provide numerous advantages. By doing so clinical staff can be kept aware of the progress being made with an autopsy of interest. Even more importantly, the final autopsy results can be more readily shared (especially when significant or unexpected findings are noted) and incorporated into clinicopathological correlation conferences and other interdepartmental teaching opportunities.

Reporting significant and unexpected findings to clinicians and presenting said findings at clinicopathological conference (CPC) both present opportunities to showcase the utility of the autopsy as a measure of patient care quality. However, the use of autopsy reports in these settings often ends at the level of academic interest or resident education without taking the next step: instituting systems-level change within the hospital. The true power of the autopsy rests in its direct application to established quality management programs in other departments of the hospital. As such, CAP accreditation requires that hospitals document the methods by which autopsy reports are used for institutional QM projects.

Even in institutions with low numbers of autopsies, individual cases can be very significant. For example, one might report an infectious disease that was diagnosed at autopsy to the infection control committee. Aggregate autopsy data has the potential to be even more useful and can be obtained with modest expenditures of time and effort. Most pathology information systems include a method of flagging cases for QA purposes (e.g., autopsies which have interesting or clinically unexpected findings). These cases can be retrieved electronically at year's end (or even more frequently for institutions with a large relative number of autopsies, such as hospitals with pathology residency programs), and a rate of unexpected or interesting findings can be established. The analysis of flagged cases could include the input of appropriate clinicians and the application of the Goldman system [18] to unexpected findings in order to determine their clinical impact. The resulting conclusions can be reported to the hospital QM office. If followed over a span of years, the rates and types of unexpected findings can reveal trends in patient outcomes categorized by diagnosis. The potential result is an interdepartmental prospective program of QA that has the potential to identify future QI projects.

Unfortunately, a frighteningly large number of hospital systems struggle to adequately incorporate autopsy data into their QM activities. Autopsy QA and institutional QI are intertwined processes such that a successful QA program also emphasizes quality improvement; that is why CAP and other accreditation bodies recognize institutional QI as an integral part of proper quality assurance in autopsy.

The Autopsy, Clinical Diagnosis, and Patient Outcomes

This section will review the past use and continued effectiveness of the autopsy as a QI tool. This will be followed by a discussion of clinical outcomes in the USA and the growing interest in improving the rate of medical errors generally and diagnostic errors in particular. The role of autopsy data in a national program of improving diagnostic accuracy will be discussed.

The Autopsy and Clinical Medicine

The examination of human remains has a long and convoluted history which has been well covered in an earlier chapter in this book and elsewhere [19], but a few points are worth mentioning in the present context. In 1844 when Carl Rokitansky became a full professor of pathology, he was perhaps the first career academic pathologist. He had never had a clinical practice. For hundreds of years before that, most autopsies had been performed as part of an ongoing clinical practice. Physicians performed autopsies to check their clinical impressions against the anatomic findings. That is to say, the autopsy served as QC on their diagnoses. Of course, there were other benefits for the medical profession, medical trainees, and society, but academic clinicians used autopsies to make themselves better diagnosticians.

The process worked. After centuries of stifling subservience to expert opinions, physicians gradually developed an objective standard against which to judge their diagnoses. It would be hard to overstate the impact on medical training and practice. As academic hospitals in France, Austria, and Germany became larger and promoted increasing specialization, most clinicians (with notable exceptions) concentrated on their patients and left autopsies to specialty-trained pathologists. However, close connections remained between hospital physicians and pathologists. Autopsies remained a sought-after means of putting nagging clinical doubts to rest. CPCs remained a valuable QM and educational tool. Hospital autopsy rates were seen as an indicator of an institution's commitment to patient care and medical education. In the 1950s about 50% of patients who died in US hospitals came to autopsy.

The dramatic decline in hospital autopsy rates in the USA and around the world has been noted, and the medical literature has offered a wide variety of explanations [20, 21]. What will not be found in the literature is any evidence that the autopsy has lost its power as a QM tool. Richard Cabot's landmark paper in 1912 [22] reaches substantially the same conclusions as the exhaustive review by Shojania, Burton, and Goldman [23] 90 years later and numerous other papers in between [18, 24, 25]: (1) autopsies reveal unsuspected, clinically important diagnoses in a significant fraction of cases and (2) physicians cannot reliably predict which of their cases will yield unexpected results. This remains true despite dramatic advances in laboratory medicine and diagnostic imaging. The authors are not aware of any data that contradicts these conclusions.

The Role of Autopsy in Improving Clinical Outcomes

It might be argued that patient outcomes in American hospitals have already improved to a point that the routine performance of autopsies is unnecessary. The USA is indeed a world leader in health-care technology and innovation, and there is much to be proud of. However, no matter how impressed Americans may be with our system of health care, it does not hold up well to comparison against other industrialized nations. In comparisons of individual markers of health-care quality (such as maternal and infant mortality), the USA ranks behind much of the rest of the developed world. On measures of overall health-care system performance, the USA ranks last in a comparison of 11 developed countries [26]. This is true despite the fact that the USA spends more on health care as a percentage of gross domestic product than any other country in the world.

In recent years, increasing attention has been focused on the quality of health care in the USA. In 2000, the Institute of Medicine (IOM), part of the National Academy of Sciences, published an influential report on deaths due to medical errors entitled *To Err is Human*. The report concluded that more than 90,000 people per year in the USA die as a result of medical errors that occur in hospitals [27]. Some authors have questioned the methodology used to arrive at this figure and suggest that the IOM figure may be an overestimate [28], but no one argues that the problem is much too large to ignore. The topic of errors and self-regulation has traditionally been a sensitive one for the medical profession. As Blumenthal puts it in his 1994 paper, "Concerning medical error and its prevention, the profession has, with rare exceptions, adopted an ostrichlike attitude. Mistakes have been treated as uncommon and atypical, requiring no remedy beyond the traditional incident reports and morbidity and mortality conferences" [29].

To Err is Human concentrated on treatment errors in the hospital. More recently the IOM released *Improving Diagnosis in Health Care* [30], a report that specifically focused on the diagnostic process. The authors found that diagnostic errors are distressingly common and that most people will experience at least one such error in their lives with potentially devastating effects. But while the authors agreed that diagnostic errors represent a large problem, they also recognized that there was no

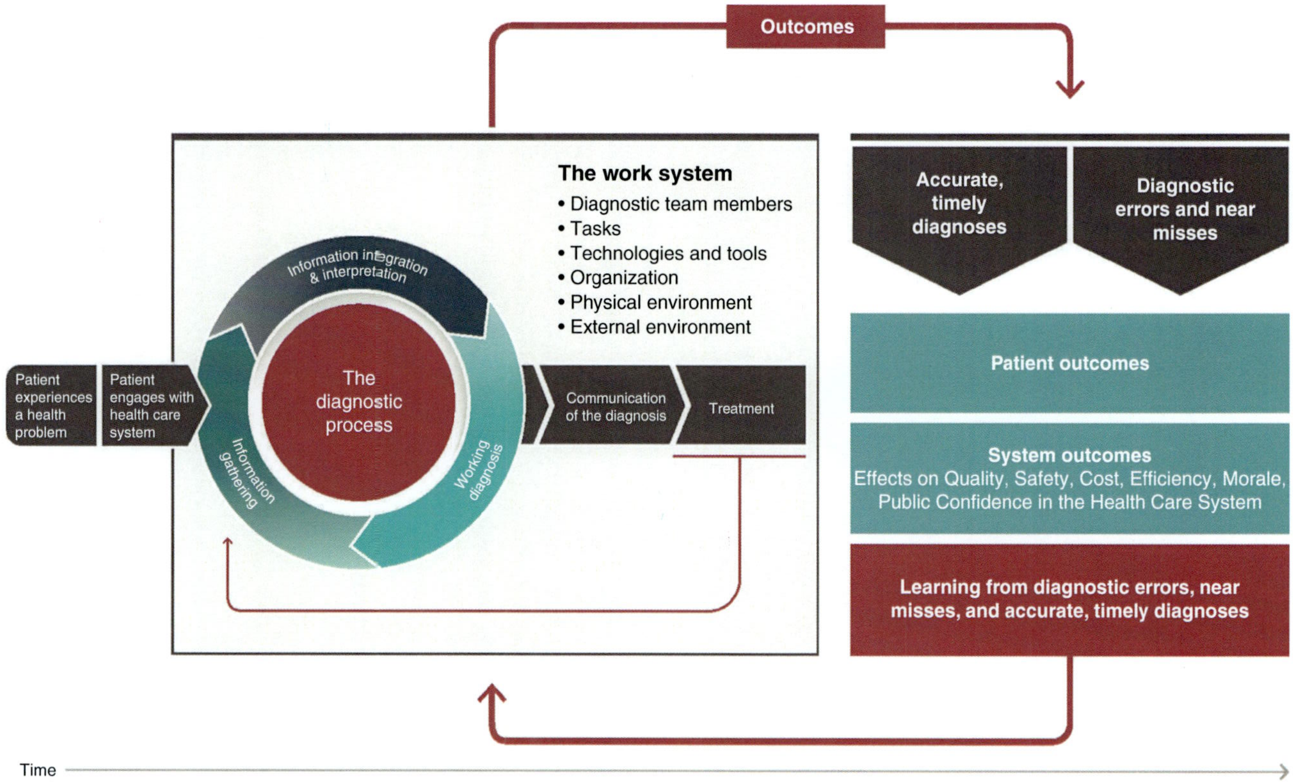

Fig. 2.2 Feedback loop of diagnostic accuracy and patient outcomes. Reliable information about diagnostic accuracy and patient outcomes (outcome loop) provides feedback to the diagnostic process (work system). Autopsy data is a crucial ingredient in the feedback loop. (Reprinted with permission from *Improving Diagnosis in Health Care*, 2015, by the National Academy of Sciences, courtesy of the National Academies Press, Washington, D.C.)

way to get an accurate sense of the scope of the problem. Any rational program of QI begins with a reliable baseline measurement, but baseline information about diagnostic errors is difficult to come by (Fig. 2.2).

Most hospitals have systems in place for identifying, reporting, and tracking treatment errors. Most do not have similar systems for identifying and tracking diagnostic errors. There is no evidence to suggest that physicians as a group are a reliable source of information on medical errors. Voluntary systems for physician reporting of adverse events have a very low yield [31, 32]. In a review of reporting systems by Levtzion-Korach, only 2.5% of reports of adverse advents were initiated by physicians. The IOM panel thoroughly and systematically searched for other potential sources of information on diagnostic error and came to two conclusions: (1) only three of the methods they examined met their criteria for providing useful information on diagnostic accuracy, medical record review, review of malpractice claims, and autopsies, and (2) none of the three was reliable enough to be used alone.

Improving diagnostic accuracy nationwide is an ambitious project, and the design of such a project is beyond the scope of this chapter and the expertise of its authors. However, a few general statements seem appropriate. If we approach this question as a QI project and apply the Six Sigma DMAIC approach (see above), the first step has largely been completed: the problem has been identified and defined. The next step would be to measure validated data in order to establish a baseline. If we accept the IOM's conclusions about methods for assessing diagnostic error, then this would involve using some combination of record review and autopsy data to measure regional and national diagnostic error rates. A baseline estimate for diagnostic error could be established. Data analysis could then yield root causes for error, and programs of improvement could be implemented and assessed for their ability to improve the diagnostic error rate as compared to the baseline. At the moment, however, the process seems firmly arrested at the "M" step.

Record Review vs. Autopsy Data

How best to use record review and autopsy data to measure error? There are advantages to both methods (Table 2.1). Record review is clearly easier to perform than an autopsy, and it has the additional advantage of including a much broader group of patients. This is particularly important since the IOM has noted that most diagnostic errors occur in an outpatient setting, which is largely beyond the reach of a hospital autopsy service. Autopsy data alone would be insufficient to establish an accurate estimate of diagnostic error.

There are, however, several important advantages to autopsy data. First, while it is true that hospital autopsies can only review a small subset of medical encounters, that subset is crucial. Hospital autopsies thoroughly review the management of seriously ill patients and provide feedback on critical diagnostic decisions. Second,

Table 2.1 Hospital autopsies and record reviews as sources of information on diagnostic error

Evaluation factor	Hospital autopsy	Record review
Health hazards	Risks of infection, sharp injuries, chemical exposures	None
Ease of use	Performed in the autopsy suite and labor intensive	Performed in an office environment
Breadth of cases	Restricted to in-hospital deaths, permission of next of kin needed, excludes forensic cases	Virtually all records are potentially reviewable – inpatient and outpatient, no special permission usually required
Cost of review	Comparatively expensive (professional time, disposable material, maintenance of morgue and equipment)	Comparatively inexpensive (professional time, maintenance of medical records)
Quality of data reviewed	Objective findings (gross and microscopic) at autopsy	Data supplied by the providers being reviewed, wholly dependent on completeness and accuracy of charting
Yield	Established record of demonstrating clinically significant unexpected findings in estimated 10–20% of autopsies	Variable but low, yield of random chart review demonstrating clinically significant unexpected findings estimated at 1%

autopsy review does not depend heavily on input from the care team. Record reviews depend heavily on the completeness, accuracy, and trustworthiness of the records, all things that cannot be assured. Pathologists depend on the medical record for orientation and direction, but the gross and microscopic autopsy findings are apprehended without any intermediaries. They are measurable and objective. Finally, it bears repeating that, as reviewed above, the autopsy yields clinically significant unexpected diagnoses in roughly 10–20% of cases. The yield of random chart review varies but has been estimated at as low as 1% [33]. In short, autopsy data provides an indispensable complement to the information obtained by record review. The question is whether the additional effort and expense of obtaining autopsy data are justified.

Cost-Effectiveness of the Autopsy as a QI Measure

In 1996, Dennis O'Leary, then president of the Joint Commission, addressed the issue of the cost-effectiveness of the autopsy as a QI measure [34, 35]. While acknowledging the benefits derived from autopsies, O'Leary stated that "The autopsy won't return to what it was in the 1950s. Ultimately, in a resource-constrained environment, the autopsy is going to have to justify itself as not only being good for quality improvement but better than other quality improvement tools" [36]. As discussed above, the autopsy is different from and complementary to other QI tools, but the question of cost-effectiveness is a valid one. The answer depends on how one examines the question.

From the point of view of the family member, the autopsy is remarkably cost-effective. At most hospitals there is no charge to the family for an autopsy. On the other hand, the autopsy, as it is currently perceived by medical insurers, is decidedly not cost-effective for the pathologist. For the purposes of medical insurance, a person ceases to be a patient at the moment of death. This means that an autopsy, in a sense, is a medical procedure performed without a patient. Private medical insurers have no interest in providing reimbursement for autopsies. Medicare and Medicaid currently consider autopsies part of the administrative mission of the hospital. As a result, reimbursement for autopsies is part of the lump sum that pathologists receive for their laboratory management duties (part A payments). This means that a pathologist will receive the same part A payment whether she performs 1 autopsy per year or 100. Compare this situation to surgical and cytology specimens for which community pathologists receive a per-case fee for professional interpretation.

Autopsies require a considerable investment in time and effort. In a survey of autopsy pathologists, Sinard concluded that the average full autopsy on an adult patient required professional work equivalent to 5.5 large, complicated surgical resections with gross and microscopic examination (CPT code 88309-26) [36]. Examination of the brain and the composition of a detailed clinical-pathologic correlation added another 1.5 × 88,309 each. The authors are aware of no other medical procedure of this magnitude that is performed in a hospital at no fee.

If looked at in the short term, the autopsy is also not cost-effective for the hospital. Again, the hospital receives no additional payment from any source for performing autopsies. There are, however, expenses: the disposable items (personal protective equipment, blades), durable items, chemicals, the cost of maintaining an autopsy suite, storing tissue and blocks, and maintaining credentialing. Faced with this stark situation, some community hospitals have understandably chosen to close their autopsy services and refer autopsy cases to larger institutions.

The evolution of QM techniques has clearly shown that there is a financial benefit to organizations that invest time and resources in QI and enormous potential expenses for organizations that do not. Using autopsies sporadically to examine small numbers of selected cases of interest is valuable as a teaching tool, but of limited utility as a statistical management tool. The goal from a QI perspective is not to find out what might have gone wrong in an individual case, valuable as that information may be. Rather the function of collecting and monitoring autopsy data in a QM setting is similar to that of a control chart in the clinical laboratory. The idea is to monitor performance, detect trends and deviations from the expected as early as possible, and intervene to correct potential problems. That is to say that from a QM perspective, the goal is not to retrospectively inspect any particular case (an exercise in QC), but rather to use data as part of an ongoing program to improve the performance of the entire system (QI). At an institutional and national level, autopsies are an indispensable part of a prospective, ongoing program of diagnostic error reduction. History and the manufacturing experience suggest that the identification and reduction of errors will lead to improved care, improved patient satisfaction, overall reduced expenses, and ultimately increased profits.

Quantity and Quality of Autopsies

In order to maximize the potential of autopsies as part of a QM program, they must be of high quality (see above section on autopsy QA), and, equally importantly, they must be done in sufficient quantity. It is difficult and statistically invalid to draw conclusions about the accuracy of diagnoses based on a sample of a few percent of hospital deaths. Authors disagree on what an appropriate minimum acceptable hospital autopsy rate is or whether or not such a number even exists. That argument is valid for considerations of medical education and training, but not for a QM program. A rational program of QI would begin by deciding on the level of confidence required of the results followed by a statistical calculation of the sample size needed to achieve that level of confidence. The authors claim no expertise as statisticians, but it is clear that most current hospital autopsy rates do not approach a statistically significant sample size. It is also worth noting that for the autopsy, as for any medical procedure, quantity is a crucial ingredient in quality. As the system is currently configured, hospital autopsies are done in greatest numbers by pathology residents and pathologist assistants. If we set aside forensic autopsies, only pathologist assistants perform a significant number of autopsies after they complete their training. Current hospital autopsy rates make it difficult for pathologists to maintain their proficiency.

An often expressed argument by pathologists against a minimum hospital autopsy rate is that there is no utility in performing autopsies in cases in which the cause of death is clear and no educational benefit will be derived. Doing autopsies just to meet an arbitrary target number, these pathologists argue, is pointless. From their individual standpoint, that argument seems valid, but ignores several crucial points. First, as shown in repeated studies over the last hundred years (see above), physicians cannot predict which autopsy cases will yield significant unexpected results. Second, those unexpected results historically comprise 10–20% of autopsies. This means that 80–90% of autopsies will yield no surprises. Put more bluntly, not every autopsy needs to be a case report. The value to the hospital of finding significant results more than offsets the time and trouble involved in obtaining the data. The clinical laboratory does not stop monitoring the results of its automated instruments simply because they rarely find problems.

It may be argued that no matter how great the theoretical benefits, from a practical perspective, the costs associated with increasing the hospital autopsy rate and centralizing the resulting data are prohibitively high. But there are a few examples of systems which maintain statistically significant hospital autopsy rates, compile national autopsy data for use in vital statistics and research, and do so with comparatively modest expenditure. The health-care system in Cuba is a good example [37]. Over 50% of patients who die in Cuban hospitals come to autopsy. Just as in the USA, hospital autopsies require the consent of next of kin. Autopsies in teaching hospitals in Cuba are a regular part of education and professional development, and the data from autopsies is maintained in a national database. The results of autopsies can be used to update and correct information on death certificates. Autopsies in Cuba are one component of a system that results in health-care outcomes that are comparable to large industrialized nations obtained at a small fraction of the cost, the very definition of cost-effectiveness.

The Future of Autopsy in QI and of QI in Autopsy

As the vignettes discussed above demonstrate, there are benefits to a conscientious QM program. The US government made liberal use of QM experts like Deming to improve the manufacturing output under the pressure of World War II. Once that pressure was removed, US manufacturers relaxed their efforts. Their Japanese counterparts did not. The rise of Japanese manufacturing again demonstrated the power of QM techniques and the risks of ignoring them. QI prevents problems, improves the quality of the finished product, engages the workforce, and is ultimately good for the bottom line. It is not sufficient to do just enough to pass inspections and remain accredited. Pathologists still feel the consequences of the 1987 exposés of commercial cytology laboratories, all of which were accredited and had at least nominal QA programs. Failure of medical professionals to effectively regulate themselves and control the quality of their work can result in external regulation, regulation which is often reactive, hastily conceived, onerous, and ineffective.

The autopsy as a QM tool does have short-term disadvantages compared to record review. But as the Ford Pinto incident illustrates, emphasizing expedience and short-term profits over the long-term quality of the product and safety of customers is not only unethical but also bad for business. The success of tissue committees in the 1950s in modifying surgical practice is a model of the sort of multidisciplinary, collaborative effort that can improve patient outcomes and can be done at hospitals of any size. It also showed that pathologists can and should play a crucial role in QI. Finally, the examples of Semmelweis and Codman show that even well-designed, well-intentioned QI projects can fail without the appropriate collaboration and institutional support.

The publication of *Improving Diagnosis in Health Care* has started an important conversation about improving clinical diagnoses and patient outcomes. The specifics of the design and implementation of a national program to improve clinical diagnosis are still in development, but several aspects of that plan are clear and germane to the present discussion. The authors of that report, after careful review of all available options, have concluded that autopsies should be one part (along with medical record review and review of malpractice claims) of the data collection necessary to establish a current baseline of diagnostic accuracy, monitor future performance, and assess the effectiveness of interventions. If autopsy data collection is going to succeed as part of an effort to improve clinical diagnosis by applying sound statistical QM principles, then the program must have several features:

1. It must be sufficiently broad in scope, i.e., the sample size must be large enough and representative enough to allow for statistically sound inferences.
2. Autopsy technical performance and reporting must be of high quality. There is currently no mechanism for training and certifying the expertise of non-forensic autopsy pathologists after residency.

3. The data from across the country must be standardized and comparable. (See sections on standardized reporting elsewhere in this book.)
4. The data must be easy to access and readily available to reviewers and decision-makers.

This will require a collaborative effort on the part of individual pathologists and clinicians as well as the vocal support of their professional societies. MQM experts should be involved in the planning phases and in the ongoing data collection and analysis. Any plan, no matter how well conceived or data driven, will fail without the administrative and financial support of hospital administrators, private insurers, government insurance, and health-care policy-makers.

The success of the autopsy phase of this program will require careful examination and rethinking of the autopsy performance and reporting processes. Generating the necessary volume and quality of autopsies may require the creation of regional autopsy centers. Coordinating the large volume of data needed will require innovative information technology solutions. Finally, there will have to be frank discussions of the costs involved. Other chapters in this book address some of these important issues.

References

1. Ross TK. Health care quality management: tools and applications. San Francisco: Jossey-Bass (Wiley); 2014.
2. Bellows B. Brief history of quality, part 1. Lean Manage J. 2015;5(2):32–5.
3. Bellows B. Brief history of quality, part 2. Lean Manage J. 2015;5(3):26–8.
4. Bellows B. Brief history of quality, part 3. Lean Manage J. 2015;5(4):40–1.
5. Wrege CD. The efficient management of hospitals: pioneer work of Ernest Codman, Robert Dickinson, and Frank Gilbreth; 1910-1918, Academy of Management Annual Meeting Proceedings; 1980. p. 114–8.
6. Marjoua Y, Bozic KJ. Brief history of quality movement in US healthcare. Curr Rev Musculoskelet Med. 2012;5:265–73.
7. Donabedian A. Evaluating the quality of medical care. Millbank Q. 1966;44(3):166–203.
8. Becker PJ, Jipson AJ, Bruce AS. State of Indiana v. Ford Motor Company revisited. Am J Crim Justice. 2002;26(2):181–202.
9. Bogdanich W. Lax laboratories: the Pap test misses much cervical cancer through labs' errors – cut-rate 'Pap Mills' process slides using screeners with incentives to rush – misplaced sense of security? Wall Street J. 1987;1.
10. Herndon JH. Ignorance is bliss. Harv Orthop J. 2013;15:74–7.
11. Semmelweis I. (translated by K. Codell Carter). Etiology, concept and prophylaxis of childbed fever. Madison: University of Wisconsin Press; 1983.
12. Nuland S. The doctor's plague: germs childbed fever, and the strange story of Ignac Semmelweis. New York: WW Norton & Company; 2004.
13. Reverby S. Stealing the golden eggs: Ernest Amory Codman and the science and management of medicine. Bull Hist Med. 1981;55(2):156–71.
14. Weinert HV, Brill R. Effectiveness of hospital tissue committee in raising surgical standards. JAMA. 1952;150(10):992–6.
15. Verda DJ, Platt WR. The effectiveness of the tissue Committee at the Missouri Baptist Hospital. Bull Am Coll Surg. 1958;43(6):449–51.
16. Verda DJ, Platt WR. The tissue committee really gets results. Mod Hosp. 1958;91(3):74–6.
17. Burton JL. Health and safety at necropsy. J Clin Path. 2003;56(4):254–60.

18. Goldman L, Sayson R, Robbins S, et al. The value of the autopsy in three medical eras. NEJM. 1983;308(17):1000–5.
19. King LS, Meehan MC. A history of the autopsy. A review. Am J Pathol. 1973;73(2):514–44.
20. Shojania KG, Burton EC. The vanishing nonforensic autopsy. NEJM. 2008;358(9):873–5.
21. Lindstrom P, Janzon L, Sternby H. Declining autopsy rate in Sweden: a study of causes and consequences in Malmo, Sweden. J Int Med. 1997;242:157–65.
22. Cabot RC. Diagnostic pitfalls identified during a study of three thousand autopsies. JAMA. 1912;59(26):2295–8.
23. Shojania KG, Burton EC, Goldman L. The autopsy as an outcome and performance measure. Evid Rep Technol Assess (Summ). 2002;58:1–5.
24. Anderson RE, Hill RB, Key CR. The sensitivity and specificity of clinical diagnostics during five decades. Toward an understanding of necessary fallibility. JAMA. 1989;261:1610–7.
25. Veress B, Alafuzoff IA. A retrospective analysis of clinical diagnoses and autopsy findings in 3042 cases during two different time periods. Hum Pathol. 1994;25(2):140–5.
26. Schneider EC, Sarnak DO, Squires D. Mirror, mirror: how the US Health care system compares internationally at a time of radical change. Commonwealth Fund, July 2017.
27. Committee of Quality Health Care in America. Kohn LT, Corrigan JM, Donaldson MS, editors. To err is human, building a safer health system. Washington DC: National Academy Press; 2000.
28. Thomas EJ, Lipsitz SR, Studdert DM. The reliability of medical record review for estimating adverse event rates. Annals of Int Med. 2002;136(11):812–6.
29. Blumenthal D. Making medical errors into 'medical treasures'. JAMA. 1994;272(23):1867–8.
30. Improving Diagnosis in Health Care. In: Balogh EP, Miller BT, editors. Institute of Medicine Committee on Diagnostic Error in Health Care. Washington DC: National Academies Press; 2015.
31. Farley DO, et al. Adverse-event-reporting practices by US hospitals: results of a national survey. Qual Saf Health Care. 2008;17:416–23.
32. Levtzion-Korach O, et al. Integrating incident data from five reporting systems to assess patient safety: making sense of the elephant. Jt Comm J Qual Patient Saf. 2010;36(9):402–10.
33. Schwartz A, et al. Uncharted territory: measuring costs of diagnostic errors outside the medical record. BMJ Qual Saf. 2012;21(11):918–24.
34. O'Leary DS. Relating autopsy requirements to the contemporary accreditation process. Arch Pathol Lab Med. 1996;120:763–6.
35. Schreuder C. Once commonplace, hospital autopsies dwindle. Chicago Tribune; 1996.
36. Sinard JH, et al. Accounting for the professional work of pathologists performing autopsies. Arch Pathol Lab Med. 2013;137(2):228–32.
37. Espinosa-Brito AD, Hurtado de Mendoza-Amat J. In defense of clinical autopsy and its practice in Cuba. MEDICC Rev. 2017;19(1):37–41.

The Future of Autopsy Reporting: Data Repository and Research Support

3

Dylan V. Miller and Billie Fyfe-Kirschner

A Brief History of Autopsy Reporting

Over the millennia that postmortem examinations have been conducted, the manner of reporting autopsy findings has no doubt evolved. Little is known about the early history, although extant records from European centers such as Padua and Vienna dating back several centuries provide a glimpse into the western tradition. In a recent review, it was noted that reports were written in *Kurrentschrift* (an archaic form of German language handwriting based on late medieval cursive writing) until the early 1800s and then in Latin script until the 1920s when typewriters revolutionized reports. Their study was possible due to storage of reports in the Vienna Municipal Archives, making the reports available for study and investigation in perpetuity [1].

In the United States, autopsy reporting was impacted dramatically by the "Flexner report" in 1910, which underscored clinicopathologic correlation as a key tenet of modern medical education. Autopsy pathology was a cornerstone of this correlative process, and the formatting of reports made accessible findings that confirmed or refuted physical examination findings and antemortem diagnoses. This was further bolstered by the Joint Commission on Hospital Accreditation requiring that at least 20% of hospital deaths be autopsied (from 1951 to 1970).

In the last quarter of the twentieth century, autopsy reports evolved to follow a fairly standard format with conserved report sections and relatively uniform content across different cases and different institutions. Increasingly, the report assumed the role of a medicolegal document. This was in part the product of standardization

D. V. Miller (✉)
Department of Pathology, University of Utah School of Medicine, Intermountain Medical Center, Murray, UT, USA
e-mail: dylan.miller@imail.org

B. Fyfe-Kirschner (✉)
Rutgers Robert Wood Johnson Medical School, Brunswick, NJ, USA
e-mail: fyfekibs@rwjms.rutgers.edu

J. E. Hooper, A. K. Williamson (eds.), *Autopsy in the 21st Century*,
https://doi.org/10.1007/978-3-319-98373-8_3

efforts by the National Association of Medical Examiners, the College of American Pathologists, and other pathology organizations [2, 3]. The reports were entirely narrative, with rhetoric and language finding a balance between the intended audiences of physicians, family members, and their attorneys.

The more recent evolutionary leaps in autopsy reporting have been occasioned by (1) increasing time demands on autopsy pathologists in both the forensic- and hospital-based settings and (2) a data-centered shift across medicine in general. Almost without exception, less time is being allotted to the practice of autopsy pathology, and pathologists are being asked to accomplish more but being given less support and fewer resources. Pathologists have had to be creative and find ways to economize in autopsy reporting. This evolution mirrors what has occurred in surgical pathology reporting, as well. As will be discussed in detail in this chapter, the emphasis is now on producing concise and "actionable" reports that possess the ability to aggregate and search data on a population level. In surgical pathology, this manifests as templated or synoptic (checklist)-based reports. The degree to which this trend will translate into autopsy reporting remains to be seen. Examples of narrative versus synoptic reporting, as applied to autopsy, are shown in Table 3.1.

Essential Elements of Autopsy Reporting

Autopsy reports are unique among all the formal communications issued by pathologists. Distinguished by their length, complexity, and exhaustiveness, these reports are the product of at least as much "art of medicine" as science. Viewed by many as the pillar of prose in the pathology laboratory and a time-honored tradition taught at great pains as part of the initiation of new pathology trainees, the construction of autopsy reports is a serious matter in this field and one invoking no shortage of opinions as to its proper execution.

The autopsy report has not been immune, however, to trends affecting surgical pathology and other reports issued by pathologists. These include a general shift toward brevity (e.g., eliminating microscopic descriptions), at-a-glance readability, and formatting compatible with digital interfaces that connect to electronic health record systems.

What the future holds for autopsy reporting is open to conjecture, but some of the salient issues pertaining to ways the autopsy report may evolve over the coming decades are the focus of this chapter.

Familiarity with the basic structure and content of present-day autopsy reports is assumed here. Readers are referred to recent excellent summaries on this topic by Koponen [3] and Fligner [4] for further contextual information on this subject.

The Narrative Versus Synoptic Report Debate

Over the past decade or so, there has been a movement in surgical pathology reporting (championed by the CAP Cancer Protocols) toward a more tabular format of "synoptic" reporting [5]. The advantages to this approach in terms of

Table 3.1 Synoptic vs narrative autopsy reports using the heart as an example

Narrative	*Heart* The heart weighs 485 g (expected 280–480 g). The pericardium is smooth. The coronary arteries are widely patent without evidence of atherosclerosis, except for focal grade 3 (of 4) narrowing in the proximal LAD with plaque calcification. There is also focal narrowing (grade 2) of the RCA. The left ventricle is mildly hypertrophied (1.7 cm, septum 1.8 cm). The right ventricle is normal thickness (0.4 cm). Cut surface shows no evidence of scar, fibrosis, or hemorrhage. The tricuspid (12.5 cm), pulmonic (7.7 cm), mitral (10.3 cm), and aortic (7.9 cm) valves are all unremarkable. The oval foramen is fused.
Synoptic	**Heart**
	Weight (in g): *485* Expected weight (in g): *280–480*
	Chamber sizes:
	Right atrium: *normal*
	Right ventricle: *normal*
	Left atrium: *mild enlargement*
	Left ventricle: *mild hypertrophy, no dilatation*
	Ventricle wall thicknesses (in cm)
	Left (freewall): *1.7*
	Septum: *1.8*
	Right: *0.4*
	Myocardial scarring: *none*
	Myocardial mottling: *none*
	Coronary stenosis (grade, out of 4) (extent, location):
	LMA: *1*
	LAD: *3 (focal, proximal)*
	LCX: *1*
	RCA: *2 (focal, mid)*
	Coronary calcification: *focal, LAD*
	Coronary stents, grafts: *none*
	Valve circumferences (in cm):
	Pulmonary: *7.7*
	Aortic: *7.9*
	Mitral: *10.3*
	Tricuspid: *12.5*
	Valve leaflets:
	Thin and pliable
	No vegetations
	Oval foramen: *fused*

communicating key pathology findings include standardization, consistency, completeness, and clarity. These translate into more "user-friendly" reports that, for example, improve oncologist efficiency in finding the parameters in the report that may guide their decision-making. They also are a boon to the creation and maintenance of registries and other clinical databases, improving the reliability and accuracy of data entry from pathology reports and even enabling the automatic export and querying of data fields, obviating the need for manual data entry altogether.

While autopsy reports are fundamentally different from surgical pathology reports, drawing analogies to this kind of transformation to a synoptic reporting style is almost unavoidable in considering the future of autopsy reporting.

Still, there are proponents of the narrative reporting style, and their arguments are sound. In contemporary (synoptic era) surgical pathology, pathologists already lament the constraints of synoptic reporting in terms of the ability to convey nuance and nonstandard aspects of a given pathology specimen. Furthermore, it is easy for important information to become buried in the "sea of data," especially when synoptic reports are lengthy, dense, and juxtapose minor/trivial and more impactful pathology findings. Both of these limitations are amplified tremendously in the extrapolation to autopsy reporting.

Truly, no two autopsies are the same, and a synoptic reporting approach to autopsy findings could jeopardize the pathologist's ability to characterize the idiosyncrasies and potentially important interplay of synergistic disease processes in a given patient. There is also the fact that it may not be possible to capture the entirety of the spectrum of possible pathologies affecting any given organ in a tidy list that is amenable to synoptic reporting. Moreover, by canonizing a list of potential common findings, pathologists may over time either forget or lose the ability to recognize other rare conditions not included in the list. Overarching this argument is a general (and justified) concern that the role of the pathologist in synoptic reporting more closely resembles that of a technician rather than a physician.

Striking the balance between efficiency gains afforded by synoptic reporting and the need for a mechanism that allows for clear communication of subtlety and complexity will be the central challenge for future autopsy reporting.

Trend Toward Uniformity Within Institutions

Like it or not (for better or worse), there has been an "organic" movement in pathology programs across the country toward adoption of dictation templates, macros, and boilerplate language in autopsy reporting. This may be an effect of the premium placed on time in pathology training, as expanding rotations and increased elective time often come at the cost of time on the autopsy service in many programs. Residents have more to do and more to learn but less time for either task. So, whether in a standardized fashion (such as macros built into information systems or official dictation templates) or through a more ad hoc approach (macros, copy-paste files, or unofficial dictation templates passed from one trainee to another), there is clearly a move toward repetition and abbreviation and away from free text or real-time narrative dictation through a microphone in the autopsy suite.

Electronic Health Records and the Drive to Data

Part of the efficiency and utility realized by electronic charting, besides eliminating illegible penmanship, is the capacity for automated note authoring assistance including prepopulating certain fields with data from other electronic health information sources. Coding and documentation of medical necessity can also be facilitated by building certain rules into report authoring and allowing digital extraction of information entered into appropriate data fields.

The possibility and potential for the future of autopsy reporting in this context is discussed in a separate heading below, but needless to say, the move toward next generation Electronic Health Records (EHRs) must be part of any conversation about the autopsy report's future.

Capturing Clinical History

Certainly, a trying aspect of autopsy report writing is the accurate portrayal of the patient's past medical history and clinical events preceding death (including vital signs, imaging findings, and laboratory values [both baseline and antemortem]). This portion of the autopsy report is typically informed by other notes and reports in the patient's chart but is presented as a more concise synopsis. Because there are so many variables in play, this is also perhaps the greatest challenge in devising a synoptic or tabular format for these data in the autopsy report.

The clinical summary serves as a critically important lens through which the more objective organ-specific findings at autopsy are interpreted. For example, a history of hypertension leads to certain expectations about cardiac and renal findings, and a history of alcoholism anticipates certain potential changes in the liver, brain, and portal circulation. So, uncoupling the clinical history data from the autopsy findings data would be problematic to say the least.

At the same time, in constructing a list of possible conditions to include in the clinical history summary, it is hard to avoid redundancy with ICD-10 and other clinical coding schemes already developed for this purpose. In some future state of EHR integration, it may be possible to rely entirely on clinical documentation and ICD coding for the information that would otherwise be re-summarized in the autopsy report clinical history section. In this scenario there may no longer be a need for a separate clinical history summary as part of the autopsy report but tying this data to the autopsy findings would still be considered critical to autopsy reporting.

One additional feature captured in some hospital autopsy reports is the explicit indication for autopsy and specific questions to be addressed. This information helps shape the clinicopathologic correlation section (if included in the report). This kind of data is theoretically amenable to codifying, since the reasons for requesting postmortem examination are relatively finite. Tracking trends in these indication data could be incredibly valuable to hospital quality programs and understanding hospital autopsy trends at a macro level.

External and Internal Autopsy Findings

Organ weights and measures are easily captured in data fields, and perhaps the most direct application of templated reporting deals with these data. As mentioned before, there is a generally conserved set of descriptive gross and histologic findings, organ by organ, that could be captured in a synoptic autopsy template. Likewise, the possible findings on external examination (similar to physical examination in living patients) could be reduced to a checklist of options. Indeed, the existing templates and dictation scripts in frequent use as part of clinical progress reports across the country reflect efforts at achieving this simplification.

Almost invariably, there is a need for an "other" category or natural language text field to capture the rare exceptions. This is important for accuracy and "free expression" of pathologists even though it may also be a potential liability to the data-oriented utility of tabular reporting, especially in the creation of registries.

Adding complexity to this is the fact that for any given gross or microscopic descriptive finding, there also exists a severity hierarchy. That is, when a finding is present, how is it best quantified? This has major implications for determining which processes were likely to be clinically significant (i.e., contributing to the mechanism of death).

While the order in which autopsy findings are reported may not be important (ultimately arbitrary and customizable in a digital environment), there may be conventions ingrained in institutions that would be important to maintain in the descriptive section of the autopsy report. These approaches include organization (1) by anatomic compartment (often in the order in which they are encountered during the postmortem procedure, for example, head and neck, thorax, abdomen, pelvis, brain, and spinal cord); or (2) by organ system, for example, neurologic, circulatory, respiratory, digestive, genitourinary, endocrine, etc.; or (3) from cranial to caudal, for example, brain, head-eyes-ears-nose-throat, neck, breast, lungs, mediastinum, heart, etc. Further details of new templates for autopsy reporting are discussed in a separate section below.

The Future of Autopsy Reporting: Why Change?

If autopsy examination is to remain an important source of data for clinicians, next of kin, communities, and institutions, it is clear that change is mandatory. Preservation of the autopsy may need a perception change as fundamental as that following publication of Morgagni's treatise "De Sebidus et causis morborum per anatomen indagatis" [6, 7]. This publication is credited with establishing modern medical practice through the identification of anatomical cause of disease and introducing anatomic-clinical correlation.

Declining Autopsy Rates

Decreased interest in this previously groundbreaking advance in medical thought and practice (the autopsy) is attributed to many factors: ability of noninvasive imaging methods to identify anatomic and some physiologic alterations, clinician confidence in these tools, elimination of minimum autopsy rate for hospital accreditation (1971), fear of litigation among clinicians, and lack of pathologist and family interest [8]. Current hospital autopsy rates are variable but average less than 10% [8].

However, the value of autopsy has not declined, with studies demonstrating that at hospital autopsy rates of even 5%, a major pre- and postmortem diagnostic discrepancy rate of almost 25% is identified. In almost 7% of these cases, identification of the missed diagnosis prior to death would have changed management and perhaps prolonged survival (class 1 missed diagnosis – Goldman criteria) [9, 10]. These data derive from reviews of 53 autopsy series over a 40-year period.

From studies like this, the statistical value of a nationwide database compiling uniformly and accurately codified autopsy data becomes readily apparent. Such data could and should drive nationwide healthcare quality metric data and research funding. In the era of quality-based medical care, the role of autopsy cannot be overemphasized. Graber argues that although autopsy is capable of identifying diagnostic errors, and indeed the impact of diagnostic errors (identification of class I errors), it is not always capable of identifying why the error was made [11]. One could argue, however, that the autopsy as a trigger for root cause analysis in cases of class I missed diagnoses should be able to supply such data at least in a significant subgroup. Performance of such a root cause analysis should be included as part of any autopsy quality assurance plan and plays a key role in patient safety.

Advancing Information Technology

For all of the aforementioned to happen, autopsy data needs to be of high quality (quality controlled), temporally relevant, and reported in a manner compatible with electronic medical records and data management systems. The narrative portable document format (pdf) files copied into a patient's electronic medical record at some temporal distance following death are not providing the ability to search relevant data fields, use data to more globally measure quality, and regionally and nationally share data [8]. Synoptic reporting using standardized and accepted formats as described in preceding paragraphs will clearly facilitate such processes.

The ADASP (Association of Directors of Anatomic and Surgical Pathology) recommends quality metrics for surgical and autopsy pathology [12]. Pre- and post-analytical and analytical variables are noted, as is the importance of having a quality assurance/quality improvement (QA/QI) plan with assessment of minimum quality standards as well as benchmarks set for improvement and a committee to oversee its implementation. It is imperative to emphasize the application of such practice to autopsy pathology. However, in the modern era of decreased autopsy rate and lack of direct monetary support for autopsy performance, many institutions do not even have a designated Director of Autopsy Pathology who can ultimately be tasked with such responsibility. National standards and synoptic reporting of autopsy would facilitate coordination of quality improvement measures across larger hospital systems as well as perhaps even nationally, in part addressing this problem. One can envision peer review of autopsy reports happening more readily in the situation of a synoptic reporting system with a separate, non-charted synoptic field dedicated to this purpose.

Impact on Education/Quality Metrics

Improving quality autopsy performance and reporting is mandatory to facilitate clinician, resident, and medical student education. Part of the decrease in autopsy rate is attributed to a decrease in pathologist interest in autopsy [8]. Some of this relates to resident autopsy exposure and education during training. The American Board of Pathology (ABP) mandates that a resident wishing to take the certification examination in anatomic pathology or anatomic and clinical pathology performs a minimum of 50 autopsies. Residents must report age group, gender, primary pathologic diagnosis, and the postgraduate year (PGY) in which they completed the autopsy [13]. This oversight assures 50 unique autopsy exposures of differing age groups (and presumably with a large enough exposure to many diagnostic categories), but the quality of such autopsy experience is much more difficult to ascertain. Nationally adopted uniform reporting standards should at least help to begin to set the minimum standard for autopsy performance and reporting and might be one way that certifying agencies such as the ABP can begin to survey quality. In addition, this move to future templated reports lends itself nicely to a coordinated and stepwise progression in assessing competency, helps clearly define the scope of what skills are necessary for residents to show independence, and documents milestone progression as residents gain more autopsy experience.

Another way to envision templated reports facilitating nationwide autopsy performance standards is to potentially tie them to quality metrics for practicing pathologists. CAP-derived physician quality measures for Medicare reimbursement incentives recommend adherence to synoptic reports as one of their quality metrics. One could envision a time when such adherence to synoptic autopsy reports is similarly proposed [14].

Development of New Templates for Autopsy Reporting

Logistical Considerations

A detailed description of the intricacies of designing database architecture is beyond the scope of this chapter, but some basic principles are helpful to review. In an electronic synoptic reporting system, a number of data field types would be needed to capture the relevant parameters. These would include defined lists (as in drop-down menus), free numeric data, free alphanumeric data, and binary selections (present/absent). The data entry interface must be customized with an eye toward ease of use and have built-in quality checks. This interface may be separate from the main report structure or may be integrated into the report itself. An example of one possible design for capturing gross data from kidney examination is presented in Table 3.2. This is constructed following principles of autopsy reporting set forth by Hanzlick et al. [2].

Once the data fields are established and populated, they may be reassorted in customized report (output) formats. These would include stylistic preferences and

Table 3.2 Synoptic data design model for autopsy gross kidney findings

Kidneys
Right kidney weight: [Numeric] g; *Size*: [Numeric] × [Numeric] × [Numeric] cm
Left kidney weight: [Numeric] g; *Size*: [Numeric] × [Numeric] × [Numeric] cm
Kidney capsule strips: [Defined list] easily/with difficulty/others: [Free text]
Kidney surfaces show: [Defined list] persistent fetal lobulation/depressed infarcts/coarse granularity/smooth granularity/smooth texture/others: [Free Text]
Kidney cut surface cortex is: [Defined list] brown/red-brown/pale brown/others: [Free Text], and [Numeric] cm thick
Kidney cut surface medulla is: [Defined list] light brown/red-brown and the corticomedullary junction [Defined list] distinct/indistinct/others: [Free Text]
Pelvicalyceal system: [Defined list] normal/others: [Free Text]
Cysts: [Binary] present/absent; [Defined list] medullary cysts/cortical cysts/both; [Defined list] right/left/bilateral; ranging from [Numeric] to [Numeric] cm in greatest diameter
Stones: [Binary] present/absent; *Stone Location*: pelvis/ureter/others: [Free Text]
Tumors: [Binary] present/absent; Description: [Free Text]
Renal artery and vein: [Defined list] Single/Dual/Multiple artery system; [Defined list] Renal artery patent bilaterally/ostial stenosis/atherosclerosis/fibromuscular dysplasia/others: [Free Text]
Ureters: [Defined list] Slender and patent bilaterally/other: [Free Text]; [Defined list] Single/Dual ureters; [Defined list] right/left/bilaterally

perhaps grouping findings by organ systems or anatomic compartment, as mentioned previously. Reports compiled solely for quality efforts, research, or monitoring purposes could also be developed using autopsy data fields. Examples could include trending lung weights (normalized to body weight) in intensive care unit deaths over time, or tricuspid valve annular diameters in patients with pulmonary hypertension compared to a reference group (or untreated cohort).

Another critical consideration for electronic autopsy reporting is the potential alterations to the report structure and format that may occur as data pass through an electronic interface to the EHR. There are generally established standards that help ensure successful passage through this process, but some validation of that protocol and careful examination of reports as viewed through the clinical EHR portal are important in ensuring success in this aspect of autopsy reporting.

One novel approach to "next-generation" autopsy reporting is detailed by Wittekind et al. [15]. They propose restructuring the elements of a conventional autopsy report into a modular format, making each section self-contained and separate. An example of how such a report might look is shown in Table 3.3. Although not their initial intent, this approach could lend itself well to database architecture.

Potential Benefits to Pathology Departments

Autopsy reports are labor intensive. The time involved in collecting and organizing the necessary information, and then in dictation, transcription, and proofing, is considerable and costly. The potential for ease of data entry and time efficiency for

Table 3.3 Complete example of a modular autopsy report format with content

<table>
<tr><td colspan="2">Module 1: Patient demographic information
Autopsy accession #: AU18–0024
Name: Jane Q. Doe
Birthdate: 01/02/1934
Date/Time of Death: 07/30/2018/23:14
Place of Death: Thoracic ICU
Date/Time of Autopsy: 08/02/2018
Ordering Physician: D. Doctor, MD
Autopsy Pathologist: R. Virchow, MD</td><td>Module 2: Clinical cause of death determination and clinical history
1a. Acute pneumonia
b. Etc.
This 84-year-old woman was admitted from her care center with dyspnea and increasing oxygen demands. Sepsis protocol was initiated, but she became progressively unstable hemodynamically and died later that evening</td></tr>
<tr><td colspan="3">Module 3: Autopsy cause of death and sequence of events leading to death
1a. Pulmonary embolism
b. Hypercoagulable state
c. Pancreatic carcinoma
2. Hypertension
The cause of death in this case is pulmonary embolism from a deep venous clot in the left leg. The underlying cause of death was pancreatic carcinoma, which is often associated with a paraneoplastic hypercoagulable state (“Trousseau” phenomenon). No evidence of acute pneumonia was seen.</td></tr>
<tr><td colspan="3">Module 4: Final autopsy diagnoses
1. Acute pulmonary embolism:
(a) Multiple thromboemboli, distal artery branches, bilateral lungs
(b) Adherent nonocclusive thrombus in left femoral vein
2. Pancreatic adenocarcinoma, poorly differentiated:
(a) Spiculated 3.2 cm mass in the pancreatic head
(b) Multiple liver metastases, all lobes, 0.2–2.3 cm
(c) Multiple peripancreatic lymph nodes
3. Right ventricular enlargement (etc.)</td></tr>
<tr><td colspan="2">Module 5: Tissue sections taken
Lungs – RUL, RML (triangular) (A1), LUL LLL (A2)
Heart – LV-I (A3), RV-L (A4), LAD (A5)
Esophagus and stomach – stock bottle (etc.)</td><td>Module 6: Ancillary test samples taken
Blood (R groin) – red top, filter spot, freezer
Urine (aspirated) – freezer (etc.)</td></tr>
<tr><td colspan="3">Module 7: Summary of microscopic findings</td></tr>
<tr><td>Block</td><td>Stains</td><td>Findings</td></tr>
<tr><td>A1–2. Lung</td><td>H&E, Gram</td><td>Thromboemboli, congestion, no inflammation</td></tr>
<tr><td>A3. Heart</td><td>H&E</td><td>Mild myocyte hypertrophy, no ischemic changes (etc.)</td></tr>
</table>

Adapted from Wittekind et al. [15]

pathologists and autopsy staff in a future state of electronic autopsy reporting is great. Savings would also be realized by eliminating transcription costs and potentially integrating images into reports (rather than handling them separately).

Quality efforts could also be bolstered by the potential for standardization and uniformity in autopsy reporting across providers as well as across different case types. The error reduction that could result from this would also save downstream time and expense correcting reports and clearing up confusion. Peer review would also be easier to perform.

Potential Benefits to Hospitals, Providers, and Families

Error prevention (or at least reduction) has been mentioned as a benefit to pathology departments already, but this also translates to improved clarity in the communication of autopsy findings to clinicians. Of course, the foremost concern of most clinicians, turnaround time, could also be improved by more real-time electronic and synoptic autopsy reporting.

Data availability for quality efforts based on autopsy report parameters could also be of tremendous benefit to clinical programs and hospital quality teams. These could be diagnosis-specific or procedure-based (e.g., complication rates). As institutions make the move toward becoming high-reliability organizations, such data could become part of a templated autopsy report under quality assurance (diagnostic error classification, safety event classification) that may or may not be a chartable component of the report but could also be searchable. Another potential benefit to institutions would be to include the results of root cause analyses and interdepartmental presentations (e.g., morbidity and mortality conferences) in portions of an electronic autopsy report that may be searchable but not reportable.

Potential Benefits to Society

Autopsy reports, collectively, contain a wealth of information that could augment and dramatically improve public health statistics, disease trend tracking, and other measures in the interest of societal good. Most current data is based on death certificate reports only and therefore is deeply flawed due to the variability and inaccuracies inherent to those resources. Death certificate data are used, despite their flaws, because they are easily accessible through computer registries. If future autopsy reporting practices were more amenable to digital codification and registry construction, the quality of information available for public health analysis would be remarkable and have potential for remarkable societal good. Some specific examples are provided in the next section and summarized in Table 3.4.

Table 3.4 Potential benefits for stakeholders from synoptic/searchable autopsy data

Stakeholder	Expectations from autopsy data (select examples)	Potential benefits of synoptic/ searchable reports
Next of kin	Identify COD	COD in separate field
	Understandable identification of disease important to NOK	Decrease autopsy TAT, highlight COD and NOK in understandable lay language
Clinicians	Identify COD in timely fashion	COD in separate field, decrease autopsy TAT
	Identify patient safety issues/ sentinel events	Separate portion of report from EMR but searchable
	Highlight clinically unsuspected findings and clinical relevance	Clinically unsuspected findings in separate field and codified as to patient impact
Pathology residents/ pathology departments	Education	Facilitates resident competency/ milestone assessment
		May lead to increase in autopsy rate and increased educational opportunities for residents
		Ease of searching may promote clinical research projects by residents
		Increases resident exposure to informatics
	Quality	Ease of peer review
		Clinically unsuspected findings help identify cases for RCA/M and M
	Cost	Potential cost savings
Institutions/ healthcare systems	Timely reports	Decrease TAT
	Identify sentinel events for interdisciplinary investigation	Separate portion of report from EMR but searchable
	Highlight clinically unsuspected findings as quality metric	Clinically unsuspected findings in separate field and codified as to patient impact, trends followed over time
	Identify trends in healthcare-associated infections	Easier to do with searchable fields
	Ensure accurate final diagnosis coding for billing purposes	Final diagnoses can be linked to ICD10 coding for billing purposes
Researchers/ biobanks	Searchable diagnoses/ demographics	Links to ICD10
	Searchable PMI/tissue storage	Separate fields for PMI/tissue storage easy to implement
Public health	National statistics for accurate COD (research funding)	Searchable COD statements make statistics in a national registry easier to create
	Patient safety (accurate identification of sentinel events and trends)	National database of sentinel events highlights trends and national measures to improve patient safety
	Quality care	Autopsy reporting can be linked to physician quality metrics

Templated Reporting and Cross-Institutional Research

Accurate and Up-to-Date Normal Organ Weight Data

The use of templated, high-quality autopsy data in a searchable format has many advantages for institutional as well as national health quality. Even something as apparently simple as normal organ weights in any given population at any given period of time may be difficult to define with certainty. Most autopsy reports cite references that are decades old and in need of updating [16, 17]. A national database of high-quality data would be invaluable for this as well as other vital quantitative measures.

Public Health/Patient Safety

Even more importantly, qualitative data such as cause of death and vital statistics are more easily validated using easily searchable data fields such as cause of death. Variable interpretation of narrative reports has been demonstrated as a cause for error in death certification. Clear and concise communication of cause of death is a vital component of any autopsy report. Similarly, disease burden statistics, which help guide national research funding, can be made more precise with searchable fields.

The autopsy plays a vital role in our national movement toward patient safety. Since the Institute of Medicine report in 1999 *To Err is Human* citing a potential 98,000 patient deaths per year related to safety errors, the emphasis on error reduction has become a major focus at all healthcare institutions, promoted by the Joint Commission [18]. The Joint Commission is focused on patient safety and making hospitals highly reliable organizations, as well as learning organizations in which individuals learn continuously, enhancing creativity and innovation. Five components of a learning institution include team learning, shared visions and goals, similar models of thought, systems thinking, and individual commitment to lifelong learning [19]. Highlighting patient safety events as opportunities for learning and process improvement is a vital part of healthcare institutions becoming learning institutions. Autopsy examination plays a vital role in the identification and classification of the most severe category of patient safety event, a sentinel event. Patient safety events are defined as an event, incident, or condition that could have resulted in or did result in harm to a patient. A sentinel event is a subcategory: a patient safety event (not primarily related to the natural course of the patient's illness or underlying condition) that reaches a patient and leads to death or permanent harm. By definition, autopsy plays a vital role in the identification of such events, and these events may only come to light following a complete autopsy. The autopsy report can assist in identifying sentinel events and should contain enough information to facilitate the multidisciplinary investigation that should follow such an event, and it should also promote institutional learning from the event. Formalized reporting that directs pathologists to think along the lines of patient safety events and to immediately recognize and report such events is vital to public health. If we do not accurately codify such events and gather precise institutional and national statistics on them, it will be impossible to identify the effects of patient safety measures at institutional and national levels. This can only be done with uniform searchable reporting models.

Translational and Other Research

Translational research can be augmented with the use of well-annotated, searchable, de-identified autopsy reports linking to tissue resources. Collaboration for access to tissue resources for rare diseases will be easier. Use of de-identified but searchable high-quality autopsy data in support of tissue repositories will be an unprecedented resource for research.

The use of standardized autopsy data when evaluating clinical trials will augment the quality of the clinical trial data. A collective review of treatment-related mortality (serious adverse events) from Europe revealed clinical-pathologic discrepancy in 46% of autopsied cases. The autopsy rate was only 10% of treatment-related deaths, attributed in large part to the lack of requirement for autopsy following death of a patient in a clinical trial [20]. Renewed interest in obtaining autopsy on study patients, combined with well-performed, searchable autopsy-derived data, should increase the quality of clinical trial data.

When national organizations, institutions, and individuals see the benefit of high-quality, uniformly reported, and searchable autopsy data, there is hope for a new era of excitement for autopsy performance similar to that precipitated by the work of Morgagni in the 1700s.

Biorepository Partnering

Laboratories faced with logistic impediments to archiving autopsy materials (slides and blocks) beyond 10 years may consider partnering with local or regional tissue biorepositories. The potential value of these materials, including to family members with possible heritable diseases, extends well beyond the 10-year regulatory time frame for storage. While preservation of nucleic acid and proteins in autopsy tissue is a valid concern (addressed elsewhere in this text), most autopsy tissues are amenable to research assays. A highly annotated tissue source (tissue linked to comprehensive autopsy reports, especially with templating) would be an attractive resource to biorepositories.

Thoughts on Next-Generation Autopsy Reporting

Utilizing information technology to take autopsy practice and reporting to the next generation is vital to the preservation of autopsy practice in the modern healthcare system. Templates/synoptic reporting/EMR linking/searchability and database sharing are all important means to this end. Templates that are well-vetted and uniformly utilized can help direct the focus of modern autopsy practice to include *patient safety/public health* (sentinel events, patient safety issues), *quality of care* (COD statements, codified clinically unsuspected findings, peer review of autopsy findings), *multimodal resident education* (system-based education/informatics education/scholarly activity, ease of competency assessment/milestone progression), and *research* (shared databases, tissue storage data).

The modern autopsy report needs to incorporate the rules of the R's to maintain its viability in the current healthcare system; it needs to be *rapid*, *reliable*, and *relevant*. Rapidity is imperative to maintain the relevance of the individual report and to maximize the usefulness of the results to institutional learning models. Reliability of reports is vital to maintain the status of autopsy results as the "gold standard." Autopsies performed superficially without an understanding of the wealth of vital information that can be shared with all stakeholders do not promote family, clinician, or institutional interest in autopsy performance. Autopsies need to be of relevance to all stakeholders. Modifying how cases are reported, with what language, and what vital data is included can be directed via nationally vetted and shared autopsy synoptic reports and databases. Considering autopsy in this fashion is also vital to maintaining its role in resident education. With so many demands on resident educational time, creatively using an autopsy service to give residents experience in informatics, system-based practice, quality assurance, and synoptic reporting is a way to increase the *relevance* of this practice to these younger practitioners, hopefully creating a group of forward-thinking practitioners who continue to take autopsy practice and reporting to the *next generation.*

As alluded to earlier, "modernizing" the autopsy report, particularly with an eye toward synoptic formatting and data extraction, represents a double-edged sword. Potential advantages are clear, but there is clearly also potential to dilute the value and utility of these reports in the practice of medicine.

Autopsy reports are inherently subjective. Standardization using templated or synoptic fields may help improve the completeness of reporting, but autopsy findings entered by pathologists are still subject to their own medical judgment. Given their length and complexity, autopsy reports are also inherently prone to errors (particularly typographic and clerical). Limiting input to a predetermined set of options has potential to improve the overall error rate. However, since there may still be a reliance on manual entry the possibility of miscoding or inadvertently selecting the wrong option also remains.

In terms of efficiency, opportunities should be sought to streamline the reporting process and eliminate barriers to its timely and accurate completion. As an example of this, the autopsy program at Seattle Children's Hospital has published their experiences using a "LEAN" approach. Not surprisingly, given the focus of this kind of analysis, they identified delays in transfers (getting tissue to histology lab, getting slides to pathologists, etc.) as well as document approvals (signing permissions or reports). Importantly they also addressed "finding time for the autopsy" by providing dedicated schedule time to pathologists and set milestone deadlines for completing provisional diagnoses, examining the brain, reviewing slides, and producing a clinical-pathologic correlation [21]. Finding additional time may not be possible in every department, but through their approach they were able to eliminate extra steps, improve report timeliness, and enhance communication with clinical teams. “Next-generation” autopsy reporting will need to be streamlined and efficiency-focused. Finally, there is valid concern that in a synoptic format report, there is no opportunity to convey the “big picture” or overall message to the family and care team. This is particularly critical when the findings could affect the health of surviving relatives or possibly alter a practice or policy in the healthcare system. There are certainly other ways for this panoramic view to be communicated besides the autopsy report, but this implication is important to consider in the future of autopsy reporting.

References

1. Winter E, Höflmayer D, Patzak B, Feigl W. Autopsy records in Vienna since Lorenz Biermayer – a complete documentation of 195 years. Wien Med Wochenschr. 2013;163:316–21.
2. Hanzlick RL. The autopsy lexicon: suggested headings for autopsy reports. In: Collins K, editor. Autopsy performance and reporting. 3rd ed. Chicago: CAP Press; 2017. p. 377–82.
3. Koponen MA. Autopsy reporting. In: Collins K, editor. Autopsy performance and reporting. 3rd ed. Chicago: CAP Press; 2017. p. 371–6.
4. Fligner CL, Miller DV. Autopsy report. In: Fyfe B, Miller DV, editors. Diagnostic pathology: hospital autopsy. Philadelphia: Elsevier; 2016. p. 106–7.
5. Srigley JR, McGowan T, Maclean A, et al. Standardized synoptic cancer pathology reporting: a population-based approach. J Surg Oncol. 2009;99(8):517–24.
6. Morgagni GB. De sebidus et causis morborum per anatomen indagatis libri quinque. Venetiis: ex Thypographia Remondiniana; 1761.
7. Zampieri F, Zanatta A, Thiene G. An etymological “autopsy” of Morgagni’s title: De sebidus et causeis morborum per anatomen indagatis (1761). Human Pathol. 2014;45:12–6.
8. Levy B. Informatics and autopsy pathology. Surg Pathol Clin. 2015;8:159–74.
9. Shojania KG, Burton EC, McDonald KM, et al. Changes in rates of autopsy detected diagnostic errors over time: a systematic review. JAMA. 2003;289:2849–56.
10. Goldman L, Sayson R, Robbins S, Cohn LH, Bettmann M, Weisberg M. The value of the autopsy in three medical eras. NEJM. 1982;301:1000–5.
11. Graber ML. The incidence of diagnostic error in medicine. BMJ Qual Saf. 2013;22:ii21–7.
12. ADASP. Recommendations for quality assurance and improvement in surgical and autopsy pathology. Am J Surg Pathol. 2006;30:1469–71.
13. American Board of Pathology Requirements for certification, Combined Anatomic and Clinical Pathology. The American Board of Pathology; 2018. http://www.ABPath.org. Accessed 13 Jan 2018.
14. 2017 QPP Reporting Codes for 8 Pathology Quality Measures. 2017. College of American Pathologists. https://www.CAP.org. Accessed 21 Dec 2017.
15. Wittekind C, Habeck JO, Gradistanac T. Proposals for standardization of autopsy reports. Pathologe. 2014;35:182–90. https://doi.org/10.1007/s00292-013-1885-8.
16. Molina DK, DiMaio VJM. Normal organ weights in men. Am J Forensic Med Pathol. 2012;33:368–72.
17. Garby L, Lammert G, Kock KF, et al. Weights of brain, heart, liver, kidneys, and spleen in healthy and apparently healthy adult Danish subjects. Am J Hum Biol. 1993;5:291–6.
18. Kohn LT, Corrigan JM, Donaldson MS, editors. To err is human: building a safer health system. Washnington DC: National Academy Press, Institute of Medicine; 1999.

19. Joint Commission AHC Patient Safety Systems Chapter. 2018. Joint Commission. http://www.jointcommission.org/assets/1/6/PS_Chapter_AHC-2018.pdf. Accessed 28 Apr 2018.
20. Penninckx B, Van de Voorde AM, Casado A. A systemic review of toxic death in clinical oncology trials: an Achilles heel in safety reporting revisited. Bf J Cancer. 2012;107:1–6.
21. Siebert JR. Increasing the efficiency of autopsy reporting. Arch Pathol Lab Med. 2009;133:1932–7.

Evolving Autopsy Practice Models

4

Alex K. Williamson

Regional Autopsy Centers

The concept of a regional autopsy center (RAC) – a center of excellence staffed by dedicated and experienced autopsy pathologists who perform and report non-forensic autopsies for hospitals, private clients, and decedents' families within a geographic region – has been advocated for since at least 1974, when Dr. Joseph Freeman addressed an audience gathered at a symposium on "The Autopsy and the Geriatric Patient" at the annual meeting of the American Geriatrics Society. Especially in geriatrics where the autopsy is vitally important in delineating physiologic aging changes from pathologic processes, the procedure's decline was (and likely remains today) a serious concern to geriatricians. Dr. Freeman pointed to the rising costs associated with autopsy and the fact that they are not reimbursed by third-party insurance payers as together representing "an outstanding factor in the neglect of the autopsy." Furthermore, as fewer individual hospitals or institutions could likely afford to maintain their autopsy services moving forward, he proposed forming RACs which "could serve the surrounding institutions with greater competence and economy" [1].

Since the time Dr. Freeman addressed his audience of geriatricians, the manner in which healthcare is delivered in the USA has drastically shifted. Relatively simple, individual interactions between patients and physicians occurring in offices or hospitals have given way to more complex interactions between patients and various specialists in regionalized healthcare systems that serve populations of people. It is reasonable to assume, then, that non-forensic autopsy services should have undergone – or should now undergo – a similar transition from many independent autopsy pathologists working in different hospitals to fewer centralized autopsy

A. K. Williamson
Department of Pathology & Laboratory Medicine, Zucker School of Medicine at Hofstra / Northwell, Hempstead, NY, USA
e-mail: awilliamson@northwell.edu

J. E. Hooper, A. K. Williamson (eds.), *Autopsy in the 21st Century*,
https://doi.org/10.1007/978-3-319-98373-8_4

pathologists serving populations of people and the health systems that care for them. RACs that are affiliated with academic medical institutions and staffed by independent, competent, and enthusiastic autopsy pathologists can provide a cost-effective way to sustain the autopsy as healthcare evolves [2].

Examples of RACs

Medical examiner offices located within or affiliated with academic pathology departments, such as presently exist in Vermont, North Carolina, and New Mexico, for example, represent some of the earliest RACs. Recently, the University of Alabama at Birmingham (UAB) published its experience developing a hybrid hospital-forensic RAC through contractual arrangements with the US Department of Veterans Affairs, the Alabama Department of Forensic Sciences (ADFS), local correctional facilities and community hospitals, and decedents' families [3]. Over the course of 10 years, the RAC performed between 215 and 374 autopsies each year and brought in nearly $2 million of income from the various contracted entities. UAB noted the following benefits of developing its RAC in association with an academic pathology department: (1) being able to expand rather than having to newly develop the requisite infrastructure necessary to run such a service, (2) being situated in a larger population center by nature of the affiliated university, and (3) maintaining access to a department of pathologists with subspecialty expertise who can provide diagnostic support in challenging cases.

Other than occasional articles advocating for RACs [4] or rare articles reporting experiences forming RACs [2, 3], there is little guidance on how to actually go about consolidating autopsy services among various practice settings in a geographic region. The College of American Pathologists in its 2003 *Autopsy Performance & Reporting* publication provided an overview of the non-forensic RAC, highlighting advantages such a center would bring to the referring institutions, the autopsy center itself, and the region the center serves, and it also summarized practical considerations that should be kept in mind when establishing a RAC [5].

The Northwell Experience

In 2011 Northwell Health (formerly North Shore-LIJ Health system) – one of the largest, nonprofit, secular healthcare systems in the USA – consolidated its anatomic pathology services including autopsy pathology into one Department of Pathology and Laboratory Medicine, with an integrated service line that spanned the health system [6]. Zucker School of Medicine at Hofstra University has been affiliated with Northwell Health since it welcomed its first class in 2011, as well. Presently, the Northwell Regional Autopsy Service (subsequently referred to in this chapter as a RAC for consistency purposes) is centralized at one of the system's largest hospitals and provides postmortem care to 16 hospitals within or affiliated with Northwell Health. The RAC is led by a pathologist with interest and expertise in autopsy pathology who is board-certified in anatomic, pediatric, and forensic pathology. Almost all of the department's nearly 30 attending anatomic pathologists, including its chairman, participate in the RAC, and 16 residents each rotate through the RAC for 3 months during their 4 years of pathology training. Additionally, premedical and medical students, clinical residents, fellows, attendings, various allied health students and professionals, and healthcare administrators regularly attend autopsies at its centralized location. Four pathologists sign out all postmortem neuropathology. All autopsies are performed by one resident working with an autopsy assistant.

Presently, about two-thirds of autopsies are performed on adult decedents of all ages, most pediatric cases are perinatal cases including third-trimester fetal losses and neonatal deaths, most autopsies include neuropathology examination, and about three-quarters of the center's case volume is referred to the central hospital from other institutions. Currently, autopsies are only performed on decedents who were affiliated with the health system, and consequently, only the technical costs associated with body transportation, autopsy performance by assistants, supplies, and histology processing are charged to the referring sites. However, a fee schedule that will include fee-for-service pricing for private clients, other institutions, and research programs is being developed as the RAC continues to grow.

The potential benefits of a RAC associated with an academic medical center, drawn upon the Northwell experience and ideas expressed in the literature [2–5, 7–9], are summarized in Table 4.1. Standardization of processes through all phases of the autopsy – from obtaining consent to incorporating autopsy results into institutional quality management programs – is perhaps the most salient benefit of consolidating a region's autopsy services in one center of excellence. The high-quality and relevant autopsy data that such standardized processes generate can re-demonstrate or confirm the value of autopsy for interested stakeholders involved with the RAC, including clinicians, researchers, and administrators. Some of these stakeholders, in turn, will consequently be more likely to refer cases to and provide financial support for the RAC. With such a center of excellence established and supported, opportunities to design and advance training, education, and research follow, including creating organized rotations with formalized curricula for pathology residents, or implementing uniform research protocols for obtaining autopsy data. Very importantly, repetition of standardized processes leads to proficiency in the involved tasks, which increases efficiency while fostering safety.

Benefits and Challenges of RACs

Arranging laboratory support for autopsy services and complying with applicable regulations are tasks that are easier and more economical to accomplish at one site rather than across multiple sites. Financial viability of a RAC can be achieved and maintained through establishing fair contractual agreements with referring institutions, organizations, and families. In the case of a RAC, consolidation of resources and economy of scale, two consequences inherent in almost any centralization

Table 4.1 Potential benefits of a regional autopsy center (RAC) affiliated with an academic medical institution

Standardization of processes	
Autopsy performance	Policies and procedures Techniques Development of standards and guidelines Access to subspecialty expertise (clinical and pathology)
Autopsy reporting	Reporting format and diagnostic terminology Clinicopathologic correlation Death certification Quality assurance
Autopsy training	Pathologists (resident, fellow, attending) Pathologist and autopsy assistants Laboratory professionals Funeral directors
Autopsy education	Premedical and medical students Resident physicians, including pathologists Attending physicians, including pathologists Allied health professionals Healthcare administrators Medical researchers Public outreach (e.g., schools, interest groups)
Autopsy quality control	Performance Diagnosis Reporting
Data acquisition, storage, and dissemination	Research Epidemiology Quality management programs
Decedent affairs	Informed autopsy consent Administration of postmortem care (e.g., funeral arrangements) Jurisdictional legal compliance Information collection (e.g., medical records) Outreach and education (families, clinicians)
Safety and compliance	
Repetition of processes by personnel leads to proficiency which leads to safety	
Establishment and maintenance of one location in compliance with applicable safety regulations	
Financial incentives	
Economy of scale	Fixed costs of facility Staffing Materials and supplies Histology and ancillary testing Decedent transportation contract(s) Compliance with regulations
Reimbursement for autopsy	Fee-for-service (e.g., family request) Contract fees (e.g., hospital, medical examiner office) Procurement fees (e.g., brains for Alzheimer's Association)
Medicolegal assistance	
Provide independent and competent assessment of quality of care for referring institutions, without perceived conflict(s) of interest	
Alleviate stress on local medicolegal death investigation systems by assisting with natural and drug overdose death investigations	

process, will likely lead to attractive pricing structures in such agreements. Finally, although hospital pathologists should always perform independent, unbiased autopsies that involve objective evaluation and documentation of facts, basing pathologists at a center that is physically independent from referring healthcare facilities can help ameliorate any perceived conflicts of interest that might exist.

Although there are many benefits to centralizing regional autopsy services, the process also presents challenges that must be addressed. And in larger urban regions, there may in fact be competition among multiple RACs, particularly where there are competing healthcare systems. Table 4.2 provides a comprehensive overview of the considerations involved in establishing and maintaining the Northwell RAC. While not intended as an exhaustive list applicable to all autopsy regionalization efforts, the table hopefully will serve as helpful reference when forming and/or maintaining a RAC.

Perhaps the most important task in developing a RAC is to establish a single nidus of contact – ideally a decedent affairs office but at least a coordinator – through which all business related to the RAC can be developed, managed, and expanded.

Table 4.2 Considerations in establishing and expanding a regional autopsy center – the Northwell experience

Logistical and legal	
Establish and staff positions (including holiday and weekend coverage)	Decedent Affairs Office (ideal), or at least a coordinator position, to control all information through one email, one phone number, and one website
	Team of autopsy assistant(s)
	Autopsy pathologists
Draft and formalize contracts with referring institutions or people	Physicians' groups Hospitals and medical centers Government agencies (e.g., ME offices)
	Families
	National research organizations
	Ancillary service support (e.g., pathology, histology, microbiology, toxicology, if applicable)
Establish policies and procedures (in accordance with local legal requirements)	Transportation of bodies to and from the autopsy center with an appropriately licensed entity (e.g., funeral home)
	Disposition of remains, including fetuses
	Disposition of unclaimed bodies
	Handling special cases (e.g., prion diseases, exhumations)
	Directing anatomic gifts to medical institutions
	Collaborating with national research organizations (e.g., Alzheimer's association)
	Reporting results to referring site(s), including integration of health information technology system(s)
	Releasing material(s) to next of kin (e.g., report, photographs, devices)
	Securing and releasing autopsy materials in medicolegal cases

(continued)

Table 4.2 (continued)

Logistical and legal	
Develop and disseminate common forms (in accordance with local legal requirements)	Autopsy information packet(s) for professionals and lay persons One autopsy consent form One decedent transportation form, to track body from place of death to autopsy center to funeral home One release of medical information form to obtain medical records One release of material(s) to next of kin form (e.g., photographs, specimens, devices)
Determine and meet local requirements (may be part of affiliated medical institution or may have to be contracted)	Sufficient and appropriate space for decedent storage Sufficient and secure storage for autopsy materials, including photographs Access to ancillary laboratory services (e.g., histology, microbiology, toxicology)
Establish and maintain professional relationships	Administration at referring site(s) Regional Medical Examiner Office(s) Regional organ donation network(s) Regional medical school(s) and graduate medical education training program(s)
Financial	
Establish and update as needed a fee schedule for provided autopsy services	
Arrange for and ensure collection of fees	
Incorporate work Relative Value Units (wRVU) for autopsy into a professional compensation model, if relevant (discussed in the next section of this chapter)	
Communication	
Produce comprehensive, clear, and correct autopsy reports	
Distribute autopsy reports to appropriate individual(s) or site(s) in a timely manner	
Engage in family meetings with clinicians, as appropriate, either in person or using information technology (e.g., videoconferencing)	
Engage in departmental, institutional, and/or system-wide quality improvement initiatives, either in person or using information technology (e.g., videoconferencing)	
Advertising	
Thoroughly and thoughtfully perform and report autopsies	
Make personal introductions to key regional personnel (e.g., hospital administrators and physicians from referring sites, medical school faculty, medical examiners/coroners, funeral directors)	
Be available to discuss autopsy results with inquiring parties (e.g., families, clinicians, administrators), either in person or using information technology (e.g., videoconferencing)	
Engage with teaching students, trainees, physicians, allied health professionals, and administrative personnel through the autopsy service	
Engage in public outreach education, including seminars or public education events	

Such an office or position should be staffed by a person with strong interpersonal skills and a sincere belief in the value of autopsy. Furthermore, most logistical processes, including drafting and executing contracts among involved parties, should be developed in conjunction with appropriate legal counsel; such legal resources may exist at an affiliated academic institution, or they may have to be developed as part of the RAC. Policies and procedures should be created for almost every step in the preanalytic, analytic, and postanalytic phases of autopsy. Their existence will not only facilitate standardization of processes, as previously discussed, but it will also enable facile handling of time-sensitive or unusual inquiries, such as donating a brain to prion research or returning a pacemaker to the requesting next of kin. Generating and implementing the use of common forms, especially the autopsy consent form, are necessary for proper and efficient functioning of any RAC.

A RAC must have well-established working relationships with medical examiner offices and organ donation networks so that timely referral into these realms of postmortem care can be made with ease. If a RAC is to advocate for the autopsy in medicine and to influence the evolution of medical education, then its pathologists should be conspicuously involved with teaching at the affiliated medical school, and there should be a formalized agreement between the RAC and the institution that encourages medical students to rotate through the RAC. Periodically reviewing and updating the pricing of services in contracts, as well as arranging for consistent and timely collection of charged fees, are two tasks that are perhaps as important as the contracts themselves. And lastly, any RAC should be led by a champion of the autopsy who is effective in oral and written communication and who will advocate for the autopsy, for the RAC, and for the patients, families, and health system it serves.

Assigning Professional Value to Autopsy Performance

Of the many reasons why the art and science of hospital autopsy remain in decline, pathologists' own devaluation and lack of championing the procedure are perhaps the most alarming and perplexing. It can be reasonably argued that the autopsy gave us pathology – and in so doing gave us medicine. But sadly, many pathologists today consider the autopsy to have fulfilled its purpose and reached its zenith as their attention focuses on more "promising" pursuits such as advanced imaging applications or molecular medicine. Moreover, it is not difficult to understand the aversion many pathologists have toward the autopsy in light of the cost containment and decreasing reimbursements which characterize medical practice today [10].

Hospital autopsy practice can be challenging and time-consuming. Reviewing the voluminous clinical record of a man with multiple comorbidities who spent months in an intensive care unit before he succumbed to presumed sepsis of unknown source or meticulously dissecting and documenting the abnormal vessels in a newborn with total anomalous pulmonary venous return are tasks that are probably considered worthwhile and rewarding to most dedicated hospital autopsy pathologists. But to the typical anatomic pathologist who must sign out and bill for a certain number of biopsies per day or to the clinical pathologist managing a busy and often resource-limited blood bank, as examples, such activities can reasonably be viewed as pointless in the absence of remuneration for their performance. Planning and thoughtfully performing a hospital autopsy take time, time that is in addition to the subsequent hours required to prepare for and present the case at interdepartmental meetings or to write up the findings from a unique and/or informative case with clinical colleagues. Additionally, as the autopsy now represents the major exposure to morbid anatomy that most pathology residents will encounter in their training, successfully incorporating autopsy pathology into educational programs also necessitates much planning and commitment by hospital autopsists.

CPTs and RVUs

The American Medical Association (AMA) has assigned Current Procedural Terminology (CPT) codes for postmortem procedures, but work relative value units (wRVUs) have not been assigned by the AMA or Centers for Medicare and Medicaid Services. Consequently, there is no way to document productivity or receive reimbursement for autopsy pathology. Conversely, because CPT codes assigned to almost all other procedures in anatomic pathology have associated wRVUs (e.g., performing gross examination of tonsils, CPT 88300, about 0.08 wRVU, or signing out a breast resection with lymph nodes for evaluation of cancer, CPT 88309, about 2.8 wRVU), pathologists engaged in these professional activities can document productivity through a perhaps imperfect but nonetheless objective metric assessment [11]. It is important to note that assigned CPT codes are constant, whereas the wRVU associated with a particular CPT code can vary depending on the year and geographic location of practice.

There have been a few clues regarding how to "value" autopsy performance in the preceding decades. In the Permanente Medical Group (TPMG), an independent corporation of physicians who negotiates and contracts with the Kaiser Foundation Health Plan – which is among the largest managed care organizations in the USA – a full-time pathologist each year was expected to perform 250 autopsies or to sign out 7500 surgical pathology cases, in the absence of additional responsibilities [12]. Similarly, the National Association of Medical Examiners recommends that full-time medical examiners ideally perform no more than 250 autopsies per year [13]. Based on these data, a full-time pathologist should perform about 250 autopsies per year, and 1 autopsy is approximately equivalent to signing out 30 surgical pathology cases (i.e., 7500 surgical cases divided by 250 autopsies = 30 surgical cases/autopsy).

The Autopsy Committee of the College of American Pathologists recently proposed guidelines for recognizing the professional work of pathologists involved with hospital autopsy [14]. Members of the Autopsy Committee were asked to equate their time spent performing a typical adult autopsy and a typical fetal autopsy to multiples of the 88309 CPT code (i.e., the code used for examination of total colectomy or mastectomy specimens), and subscribers to the Committee's Autopsy Pathology Education Program were asked to report how long it took them to perform a typical adult and a typical fetal autopsy. The committee members' responses regarding time spent performing autopsies correlated with those of the program subscribers. Furthermore, the committee's proposed guidelines for how many multiples of CPT 88309 constitute the elements of performing a typical adult autopsy and a typical fetal autopsy were congruent with scant contemporaneous data in the literature regarding the effort invested in performing autopsies.

As there is great variability in autopsy practice among pathologists and institutions, these guidelines are best used as a benchmark that can and should be modified to accommodate diverse hospital autopsy practices. Members of the Society for Pediatric Pathology, for example, recognize that competent perinatal autopsies usually require more time and effort than is usually invested in examining the "typical" stillborn fetus encountered by many pathologists working outside of a dedicated pediatric care setting [15]. A recent study that surveyed pediatric pathologists performing fetal, perinatal, and pediatric autopsies also demonstrated that such autopsies – which often require complex dissections or additional ancillary testing – require additional time and therefore modified valuation with existing CPT codes [16].

An Example of Assigning Value

At Northwell, slight modifications to these proposed CPT guidelines for autopsy performance have been made. For example, complex fetal, neonatal, and pediatric autopsies are often performed by an attending pediatric pathologist with the assistance of a resident pathologist. These cases often involve complicated medical issues and/or complex dissections, audiences of medical students and clinicians often attend these autopsies, and these cases are almost always presented at interdepartmental morbidity and mortality conferences which require substantial preparation time on the part of the pathologists. On the whole, however, the Northwell Department of Pathology & Laboratory Medicine, which encompasses all subspecialties of pathology across the age spectrum, aligns fairly well with the proposed valuations from the Autopsy Committee of the College of American Pathologists and the Society for Pediatric Pathology. All currently available suggested valuations for measuring professional activity associated with adult, pediatric, and perinatal autopsies performed in hospitals, including Northwell's modifications, are summarized in Table 4.3.

Over the past 3 years, the Northwell RAC adopted these suggested valuations (with slight modifications as described above and noted in Table 4.3) to quantify autopsy work performed by attending pathologists in the department. The quantified work was then translated using prevailing wRVU scales for the region (currently 88309 = 2.8 wRVU), and the corresponding value of professional time dedicated to autopsy was incorporated into each pathologist's annual wRVU totals. The wRVU totals were then used in various departmental value-based determinations. Over the past 3 years, the total wRVU accrued on the Northwell RAC by attending pathologists aggregated to 5,796 wRVU in 2015, 7,576 wRVU in 2016, and 5,790 wRVU in 2017. These annual wRVU amounts are comparable to those of a full-time equivalent academic pathologist using presently available valuation methodology [11]. It is clear that autopsy needs to be considered and valued as is any other anatomic pathology specialty in today's subspecialized practice environment.

Table 4.3 Assigning professional value to autopsy performance

	CPT (multiples of 88309)			RVU (88309 = 2.8 RVU)		
	CAP	SPP	Northwell	CAP	SPP	Northwell
Adult total	**8.5**	N/A	**8.5**	**23.8**	N/A	**23.8**
Autopsy	5.5		5.5	15.4		15.4
Neuropathology	1.5		1.5	4.2		4.2
Clinicopathologic discussion	1.5		1.5	4.2		4.2
Pediatric total	N/A	**15.7**	**12.0**	N/A	**43.96**	**33.6**
Autopsy		9.9	8.25		27.72	23.1
Neuropathology		2.5	1.5		7	4.2
Clinicopathologic discussion		3.3	2.25		9.24	6.3
Neonate total	**6.0**	**9.7**	**11.0**	**16.8**	**27.16**	**30.8**
Autopsy	4.0	5.8	8.25	11.2	16.24	23.1
Neuropathology	0.5	1.6	0.5	1.4	4.48	1.4
Clinicopathologic discussion	1.5	2.3	2.25	4.2	6.44	6.3
Fetus >20 weeks total[a]	**6.0**	**9.7**	**6.0**	**16.8**	**27.16**	**16.8**
Autopsy	4.0	5.8	4.0	11.2	16.24	11.2
Neuropathology	0.5	1.6	0.5	1.4	4.48	1.4
Clinicopathologic discussion	1.5	2.3	1.5	4.2	6.44	4.2
Fetus <20 weeks total[a]	**6.0**	**5.7**	Billed as surgical pathology specimen (1 × 88309)	**16.8**	**15.96**	Billed as surgical pathology specimen (1 × 88309)
Autopsy	4.0	3.6		11.2	10.08	
Neuropathology	0.5	0.7		1.4	1.96	
Clinicopathologic discussion	1.5	1.4		4.2	3.92	

N/A = not applicable
CAP = College of American Pathologists; data from Ref. [14]
SPP = Society for Pediatric Pathology; data from Ref. [16]
[a]At Northwell: complex fetus >20 weeks treated as neonate; complex fetus <20 weeks treated as fetus >20 weeks

The Autopsy in Medical Malpractice Litigation

Among many potential factors contributing to declining autopsy rates since the 1940s is a perception among clinicians – and one that is probably propagated by pathologists, as well – that autopsy performance increases the likelihood of malpractice litigation and/or will corroborate physician culpability in such litigation. Today's autopsy pathologists must have at least a working knowledge of the medical malpractice landscape in which their clinical colleagues practice. Such knowledge hopefully will empower autopsy pathologists to best serve patients, clinicians, and healthcare systems through careful, competent, and unbiased performance and reporting of postmortem examinations.

Errors in judgment, diagnosis, and/or technique have characterized and will continue to characterize the human practice of medicine. However, since the turn of the century, there has been increased focus on addressing and decreasing the incidence of error and adverse events in medicine [17, 18]. In general, medical malpractice claims usually arise following adverse events, of which there are two types: non-preventable and preventable adverse events. Preventable adverse events understandably are a serious concern in today's healthcare environment. Estimated numbers of deaths arising from preventable adverse events are comparable to mortality rates from various natural diseases or conditions in many countries including China [19], the USA [17, 20], the UK [21], and Germany [22].

Overview of Medical Malpractice

In medical malpractice proceedings, a plaintiff is the person or party who initiates the lawsuit – usually the next of kin in cases of autopsy – and the defendant is the person or party against whom the lawsuit is brought, usually a doctor or healthcare institution. To establish liability in medical malpractice, a plaintiff must generally prove (1) that duty inherent in a doctor-patient relationship was established; (2) that a breach of that duty, defined by failure to exercise or meet the generally accepted standard(s) of care, occurred; and (3) that, to a reasonable degree of medical certainty, the breach of duty was the proximate cause of injury or death. There are many reasons why a plaintiff may decide to pursue litigation, but it has been documented that a lack of open, clear, and honest communication, inadequately acknowledging the pain and suffering caused by an adverse event, and not demonstrating a willingness to learn and improve from a mistake all represent factors that are associated with patients suing physicians [23, 24].

A recent study examining malpractice claims among physicians who were covered by a national professional liability insurer paints a useful portrait of the medical malpractice landscape among various specialties in the USA [25]. Select data from the study is adapted and summarized in Table 4.4. Overall, nearly 7.4% of physicians faced a malpractice claim each year, whereas only 1.6% of physicians were involved in a claim that resulted in a payment being made to the plaintiff (i.e., an indemnity payment). Certain "high-risk" specialties (including neurosurgery, cardiothoracic surgery, and general surgery) were more likely to face a malpractice claim, but these specialties tended not to make indemnity payments. On the contrary, other "low-risk" specialties (including pathology, family practice, and pediatrics) were less likely to face a malpractice claim, but these specialties tended to make indemnity payments. The mean and median indemnity payments across all specialties were around \$270,000 and \$110,000, respectively, with the skewed distribution reflecting few very large payments. For example, four specialties – obstetrics and gynecology, pathology, anesthesiology, and pediatrics – made large indemnity payments exceeding \$1 million, but such large sums only accounted for 1% of all payments analyzed in the study.

Table 4.4 Proportion of US physicians facing malpractice claim with mean and median malpractice payment amounts among representative specialties

Specialty	% Physicians with a malpractice claim (annual)	% Physicians paying a claim to a plaintiff (annual)	Mean value of payment made to a plaintiff (multiples of $10,000)	Median value of payment made to a plaintiff (multiples of $10,000)
Neurosurgery	17.5–20	2.5–5	30–35	20–25
Thoracic/cardiovascular	17.5–20	2.5–5	25–30	15–20
General surgery	15–17.5	2.5–5	25–30	15–20
Orthopedic surgery	12.5–15	2.5–5	25–30	10–15
Obstetrics and gynecology	10–12.5	2.5–5	35–40	15–20
Internal medicine	7.5–10	0–2.5	30–35	15–20
Emergency medicine	7.5–10	0–2.5	15–20	5–10
All physicians	**7.4**	**1.6**	**27**	**11**
Anesthesiology	5–7.5	0–2.5	25–30	5–10
Pathology	5–7.5	0–2.5	35–40	15–20
Family practice	5–7.5	0–2.5	25–30	10–15
Pediatrics	2.5–5	0–2.5	50–55	15–20

Adapted from figures 1 and 3 in Jena et al. [25]

The authors calculated that physicians face a high cumulative risk of encountering at least one malpractice claim during their careers. Nearly 75% and 99% of physicians in "low-" and "high"-risk specialties, respectively, will face a malpractice claim by age 65 years, and nearly 19% and 71% of physicians in "low-" and "high"-risk specialties, respectively, will make an indemnity payment. Physicians, particularly those practicing in the "higher-risk" surgical specialties, rightfully perceive that they will face malpractice litigation. However, an important observation in this study was that across specialties most medical malpractice claims did not result in payments being made to plaintiffs. This "good news" must be tempered with the reality that medical malpractice litigation can take a toll on physicians' emotions, finances, and reputation, regardless of its outcome.

Role of Autopsy in Medical Malpractice: The USA Experience

Literature meaningfully evaluating the role that autopsy plays in malpractice litigation is limited. A retrospective review of appeals court decisions regarding alleged malpractice cases in the USA is perhaps the most frequently referenced publication dealing with the issue [26]. The authors reviewed records of malpractice litigation adjudicated in state appellate courts between 1970 and 2000. The oft-cited finding from this study, presented in Table 4.5, is that even when autopsy findings were

Table 4.5 USA experience with autopsy in alleged malpractice cases

		Malpractice verdict	
Autopsy findings favor	Total cases	Yes	No
Plaintiff	49	39% (19)	61% (30)
Neither	14	21% (3)	79% (11)
Defendant	19	0% (0)	100% (19)

Adapted from Fig. 4 in Bove and Iery [26]

interpreted by the authors to have favored the plaintiff, the defendant physicians were exonerated of malpractice in the majority of cases. In other words, performance of an autopsy did not correlate with physicians being convicted of malpractice in this study.

Careful reading of the article reveals additional observations that shed brighter light on the role of autopsy in medical malpractice. All reviewed cases included the performance of an autopsy, and overall, findings favoring the defendant physician outnumbered the findings favoring the plaintiff by a 3:1 margin. Moreover, while autopsy confirmed clinical diagnoses in nearly a third of the cases (27/99), major discrepancies between antemortem and postmortem diagnoses were revealed in just over half of the cases (54/99). And although the authors considered most of these postmortem diagnoses (40/54) to have been potentially treatable in life, the majority of defendants were acquitted of malpractice in the original trials. Finally, 8 of 13 physicians convicted of malpractice in their original trial were acquitted of malpractice in their appeal process when autopsy confirmed the clinical diagnoses, and astonishingly, 32 of 36 physicians convicted of malpractice in their original trial were acquitted of malpractice in their appeal process even though the cause of death determined at autopsy had not been recognized in life.

Based on their findings, the authors suggest there is no relationship between accuracy of clinical diagnoses as revealed by autopsy and an unfavorable outcome for defendant physicians in malpractice litigation. For instance, findings of medical negligence that were upheld on appeal (19 cases) were all related to standard of care issues and not to the autopsy findings, even though in over half of these cases (10/19) there were discrepant antemortem and postmortem diagnoses. As the authors state, "...medical perfection, which is unattainable in any event, is not the standard of care." Moreover, the authors considered postmortem examinations that either confirmed antemortem diagnoses or, more often, revealed major unexpected findings that could not have reasonably been acted upon while the patient was alive, important in acquitting 17 defendant physicians initially convicted of malpractice.

Minor additional findings at autopsy were usually rendered irrelevant as opposing expert witnesses disagreed about their significance. No unequivocal cause of death was determined at autopsy in nearly 10% of the cases, including perinatal and postoperative deaths, but the majority of physician defendants involved in these cases were acquitted of malpractice. Interestingly, in 16 malpractice trials in which no autopsy had been performed (which served as "control" cases), the ratio of outcomes favoring either plaintiff or defendant physicians was similar to those in the study group, corroborating the conclusion that autopsy does not necessarily lead to adverse decisions for defendant physicians involved in malpractice litigation.

Role of Autopsy in Medical Malpractice: The International Experience

In recent years the international community has increasingly shared its experience with the role of autopsy in medical malpractice litigation [19, 22, 27]. In these studies, cases suspected of medical malpractice were evaluated by the relevant medicolegal pathology institution rather than by hospital autopsy pathologists. Similar to the experiences reflected with appellate court decisions in the USA, in Germany and Italy the majority of physicians involved with malpractice litigation were exonerated of the charges brought against them in cases in which an autopsy had been performed. When malpractice was confirmed in Germany, autopsy did not establish causality in most cases, whereas when malpractice was confirmed in Italy, autopsy established causality in a majority of cases.

In China the situation appears to be slightly less favorable for defendant physicians in general, with nearly half of all cases of suspected malpractice being confirmed when an autopsy had been performed. Moreover, discrepancies between antemortem and postmortem diagnoses were also associated with malpractice more commonly being confirmed in China, although when there was an indeterminate diagnostic discrepancy, malpractice was more commonly negated. Reasons for the reported discrepancy between China and the western countries probably reflect a variety of factors, including a younger patient population referred for malpractice proceedings in China (mean age of 31 years in China, mean age around 59 years in Italy, modal age range 71–80 in Germany), a higher incidence of suspected malpractice in China over the study period, and the fact that many cases referred for medicolegal evaluation in China reflect more complex cases that were not initially resolved by arbitration.

Recommended Practices in Hospital Autopsy Pathology

In their review of the US appellate court records discussed above, the authors also noted problematic issues relating to autopsy performance and reporting as well as death certification that affected the appeals process in nearly 20% (18/99) of the examined cases, including those that were reversed on appeal [28]. Autopsy pathologists should always perform and report postmortem examinations in a complete, careful, and consistent manner. Furthermore, autopsy pathologists should encourage clinicians to incorporate provisional autopsy findings into death certifications and to amend those death certifications as necessary in light of final autopsy findings.

Although most significant postmortem diagnoses are macroscopically evident by the end of dissection, histology can provide, modify, or confirm the cause of death in a substantial number of cases, especially in hospital-based, non-forensic deaths. For example, significant pulmonary or hepatic pathology can be missed by relying only on macroscopic examination of these organs, and there is poor agreement between the degree of coronary artery stenosis as assessed by macroscopic and histologic methods [29]. Diligent examination of autolyzed tissue, with assistance of special stains as necessary, must always be performed, as pathologies such as fibrosis and hemosiderosis can be diagnosed in almost every stage of postmortem decomposition, and such diagnoses can have important diagnostic or familial relevance (e.g., cirrhosis or hemochromatosis, respectively).

As it's very unlikely that the legal fate of a given autopsy will be known by a pathologist at the time of postmortem examination, it is advisable to approach every autopsy as though it will have medicolegal implications. Listed below are some recommended practices (based on the author's experience and the literature [28, 29]) for pathologists to consider when performing and reporting autopsies, so that objective data and not subjective speculation are on trial in potential medical malpractice proceedings.

- Be aware of specific clinical concerns or questions before beginning an autopsy, and adequately address such issues during the autopsy and in the resulting report (e.g., venous thromboembolism, specimens needed or requested for toxicology).
- Document all pathology, regardless of its lethal potential, and objectively describe relevant positive and negative macroscopic and microscopic features (don't just focus on the cause of death!).
- Adequately document and sample lesions for assessment of chronicity (e.g., hemorrhages, thrombi and emboli, infarcts) so that correlation with a clinical sequence of events can later be performed, if necessary.
- In accordance with hospital policy, collect, preserve, and appropriately maintain the integrity of specimens for toxicology or other special testing.
- Always submit appropriate specimens for histology, including at least sections of the heart, lungs, liver, kidneys, stenotic coronary arteries, and any macroscopically abnormal tissue; neuropathologic histology should be submitted, as well, when indicated.
- Keep representative sections of all examined organs and tissues in a stock jar, including a block of the cardiac conduction system if the heart base is not routinely retained.
- Issue quality autopsy reports in a timely fashion, and amend final autopsy reports as necessary (e.g., if new clinical or laboratory testing information becomes available).
- Incorporate relevant clinical history into the final autopsy report to allow for independent review of and conclusions to be drawn from the final report.
- Include a cause of death statement, when relevant, in the final autopsy report in a style that is compatible with local death certification practices.
- Review and rectify antemortem and postmortem diagnostic discrepancies with the clinician, if possible, or at least address the discrepancies in the autopsy summary, before finalizing the autopsy report.
- Ensure the final autopsy report contains no discrepancies or disagreements across its various sections (particularly the final diagnoses, gross description, and microscopic findings sections).
- Ensure autopsy reports are free of grammatical and spelling errors (remember – sloppy autopsy reporting suggests sloppy autopsy performance and sloppy autopsy conclusions).

Thoughts on the Future of These Evolving Autopsy Practices

This chapter has reviewed three evolving facets of modern (non-forensic) autopsy practice – consolidating autopsy services in regional centers of excellence, assigning professional value to autopsy performance, and promulgating reasonable expectations for the role of autopsy in medical malpractice litigation. For a long time, practitioners of the autopsy served families, physicians, and hospitals in a relatively simple and individualized context. But now autopsy pathologists must adapt their practice to serve these same parties in complex, integrated health systems that are keenly interested in optimizing patient outcomes in a value-based manner.

Regional Autopsy Centers

Autopsy pathology must be recognized and supported as is any other subspecialty within pathology. Concentrating and developing autopsy resources and expertise within regional autopsy centers (RACs) will effectively achieve such a goal. Although RACs have been promoted in the literature for decades, few have emerged in recent years. It is time to acknowledge that RACs are the future of autopsy pathology and to act accordingly. RACs should be established in all health systems, either as free-standing institutions or within one of the system's existing hospitals. RACs need to be staffed by dedicated pathologists who care about postmortem care, who are competent in autopsy pathology, who are capable educators, and who will champion the autopsy. Such autopsy pathologists will have a twofold effect on autopsy pathology: first, they will provide competent autopsy pathology services in the regions they serve, and second, they will inspire and instruct the next generation of autopsy pathologists.

Most of today's attending pathologists received only a few months of autopsy pathology training in residency, which was likely of variable quality. Presently, completing a forensic pathology fellowship is almost the only way to receive advanced training in autopsy pathology, and most graduates of forensic pathology fellowships understandably go on to serve as medical examiners. Fellowships in autopsy pathology need to be created and supported, and RACs provide a logical place for such graduate medical education programs to reside. A RAC couples large case volume with professional expertise in all aspects of autopsy performance and reporting, resulting in a rich experiential and educational program for the autopsy pathology fellow. Access to the large amount of aggregate data available at a RAC would allow for myriad research endeavors to be pursued by the fellow, as well, enhancing the fellow's development while promoting autopsy pathology scholarship. Finally, as a RAC is likely to be affiliated with at least one academic medical institution within the region it serves, the fellow would be able to engage and develop skills in all levels of education. Establishing RACS and then using them to train the next generation of autopsy pathologists represent vital steps as autopsy pathology moves forward.

Establishing and supporting RACs, let alone autopsy pathology fellowships, requires funding. Initially, RACs are likely to pay for themselves as the savings generated from closing and consolidating individual autopsy services within a region can be concentrated in a RAC through thoughtful contractual arrangements. As a RAC succeeds in producing high-quality autopsy data in an efficient and cost-effective manner, the data can then be used to demonstrate a benefit to the region the RAC serves. Then relevant stakeholders – including clinicians and administrators – will likely invest in the RAC and thereby allow its service, education, and research endeavors to grow.

RACs that incorporate forensic pathology services can play a vital role in addressing this country's critical shortage of resources dedicated to adequate medicolegal death investigation. In fact, the Scientific Working Group on Medicolegal Death Investigation (SWGMDI) has outlined plans for constructing, staffing, and financing RACs to address this problem [30]. In the University of Alabama (UAB) experience, for example, autopsies in suspected cases of natural death or accidental drug overdose were performed at UAB with appropriate forensic oversight, thereby freeing up medical examiners to concentrate their resources on other forensic death investigations. As many jurisdictions around the country face increasing drug overdose deaths [31], the role of RACs in assisting medicolegal death investigation in this country is likely to become more important in the years ahead.

Assigning Value to Autopsy

Before relevant stakeholders outside of pathology even consider paying for autopsies, pathologists and pathologists' organizations must themselves acknowledge the value of autopsy through action. Over the past 3 years in the Department of Pathology and Laboratory Medicine at Northwell, documenting and incorporating wRVU from the autopsy service into each attending pathologist's annual productivity assessment have been well received by the department's faculty. The pathologists universally appreciate being recognized for their autopsy work, and the chief of service has subjectively noted increased faculty engagement in resident autopsy education as well as improved quality of autopsy reporting. Such outcomes continue to be monitored and will objectively be assessed and reported in the future. Hopefully, other pathology departments will adopt, modify, and share their experiences with documenting and assigning professional value to autopsy pathology. Only with such aggregate data can valid proposals for reimbursement be advanced, so that autopsy pathology can ultimately receive appropriate compensation.

Although quantifying the value of autopsy in this fashion might potentially open the door to reimbursement for the procedure down the road, in the USA there remains no specific governmental reimbursement for hospital autopsies from either Medicare Part A (hospital insurance program) or Part B (supplementary medical insurance for physician services) payments. There is hope, however, that autopsy might one day be directly financed by a third-party payor such as the government, as the most recent USA Institute of Medicine report recommended "... funding for a designated subset of health care systems to conduct routine postmortem examinations on a representative sample of patient deaths" [18]. Even some insurance companies have acknowledged that autopsy could be reimbursed if it demonstrated value to an insured population [2]. For this dream to become a reality, though, the autopsy must first be appropriately valued by its practitioners, and then we can serve as advocates for having autopsy adequately funded.

Autopsy in the Medical Malpractice Environment

Finally, in today's healthcare environment – which is characterized by evidence-based medicine, patient-centered care, and cost-effectiveness – the autopsy will remain relevant if it helps optimize patient and health system outcomes through assuring the quality of healthcare. Always performing complete, consistent, and competent postmortem examinations in an objective and unbiased manner will ensure a productive and appreciated engagement in this endeavor. And as preventable adverse events will undoubtedly continue to occur in medicine – given that human nature is inherent in the practice of medicine – autopsy pathologists must prepare for and embrace their role as autopsy experts in legal proceedings involving non-forensic deaths.

The only aspects of a medicolegal case which autopsy pathologists can control are the thoughtfulness and thoroughness with which they perform and report their autopsies. It has been long recognized that well-performed and reported autopsies help "… eliminate suspicion …provide reassurances to families … substitute facts for conjecture … construct a better defense … reduce the number of claims …and improve the quality of care" [32]. Autopsy pathologists who appreciate such far-reaching consequences of a well-performed and well-reported autopsy, and who are able to meaningfully engage in the medicolegal realm, will help ensure that autopsy pathology remains an integral component of healthcare moving forward.

References

1. Freeman JT. The autopsy in geriatrics. J Am Geriatr Soc. 1975;23(1):1–10.
2. Trelstad RL, Amenta PS, Foran DJ, Smilow PC. The role for regional autopsy centers in the evaluation of covered deaths. Survey of opinions of US and Canadian chairs of pathology and major health insurers in the United States. Arch Pathol Lab Med. 1996;120(8):753–8.
3. Atherton DS, Reilly S. The regional autopsy center: the University of Alabama at Birmingham experience. Am J Forensic Med Pathol. 2017;38(3):189–92.
4. Geller SA. Who will do my autopsy? Arch Pathol Lab Med. 2015;139(5):578–80.
5. Baker PB. Chapter 9: non-forensic regional autopsy centers. In: Collins KA, Hutchins GM, editors. Autopsy performance & reporting. Northfield: College of American Pathologists; 2003. p. 75–9.
6. Groppi DE, Alexis CE, Sugrue CF, et al. Consolidation of the North Shore-LIJ health system anatomic pathology services: the challenge of subspecialization, operations, quality management, staffing, and education. Am J Clin Pathol. 2013;140(1):20–30.
7. Hutchins GM. Whither the autopsy? ... to regional autopsy centers. Arch Pathol Lab Med. 1996;120:718.

8. Horowitz RE, Naritoku WY. The autopsy as a performance measure and teaching tool. Hum Pathol. 2007;38(5):688–95.
9. Liao JM, Singh H. Reviving the autopsy as a diagnostic error–reduction tool. Lab Med. 2013;44(2):186–90.
10. Dark Daily. Tough times ahead for anatomic pathology as group revenue declines and pathologists' incomes drop due to payer price cuts, narrow networks, and claims denials.18 Jan 2017. https://www.darkdaily.com/tough-times-ahead-for-anatomic-pathology-as-group-revenue-declines-and-pathologists-incomes-drop-due-to-payer-price-cuts-narrow-networks-and-claims-denials-118/. Accessed 21 Apr 2018.
11. Ducatman BS, Parslow T. Benchmarking academic anatomic pathologists: the Association of Pathology Chairs Survey. Acad Pathol. 2016;3:2374289516666832.
12. Haber SL. Kaiser Permanente. An insider's view of the practice of pathology in an HMO hospital-based multispecialty group. Arch Pathol Lab Med. 1995;119(7):646–9.
13. National Association of Medical Examiners. Forensic autopsy performance standards. 2012. https://netforum.avectra.com/public/temp/ClientImages/NAME/3c58b363-0fa6-42cc-9f71-d2c5c0790cb1.pdf. Accessed 21 Apr 2018.
14. Sinard JH, Autopsy Committee of the College of American Pathologists. Accounting for the professional work of pathologists performing autopsies. Arch Pathol Lab Med. 2013;137(2):228–32.
15. Taylor GP, Faye-Petersen OM, Ernst L, et al. Small patients, complex challenging cases: a reappraisal of the professional efforts in perinatal autopsies. Arch Pathol Lab Med. 2014;138:865–8.
16. Pacheco MC, Reed RC. Pathologist effort in the performance of fetal, perinatal, and pediatric autopsies: a survey of practice. Arch Pathol Lab Med. 2016;141:209–14.
17. Kohn LT, Corrigan J, Donaldson MS. To err is human: building a safer health system. Washington, DC: National Academy Press; 2000.
18. National Academies of Sciences Engineering and Medicine. Improving diagnosis in health care. Washington, DC: The National Academies Press; 2015.
19. He F, Li L, Bynum J, et al. Medical malpractice in Wuhan, China: a 10-year autopsy-based single-center study. Medicine (Baltimore). 2015;94(45):e2026.
20. James JT. A new, evidence-based estimate of patient harms associated with hospital care. J Patient Saf. 2013;9(3):122–8.
21. Hogan H, Healey F, Neale G, et al. Preventable deaths due to problems in care in English acute hospitals: a retrospective case record review study. BMJ Qual Saf. 2012;21(9):737–45.
22. Madea B, Preuss J. Medical malpractice as reflected by the forensic evaluation of 4450 autopsies. Forensic Sci Int. 2009;190(1–3):58–66.
23. Vincent C, Young M, Phillips A. Why do people sue doctors? A study of patients and relatives taking legal action. Lancet. 1994;343(8913):1609–13.
24. Levinson W, Roter DL, Mullooly JP, Dull VT, Frankel RM. Physician-patient communication. The relationship with malpractice claims among primary care physicians and surgeons. JAMA. 1997;277(7):553–9.
25. Jena AB, Seabury S, Lakdawalla D, Chandra A. Malpractice risk according to physician specialty. N Engl J Med. 2011;365(7):629–36.
26. Bove KE, Iery C, Autopsy Committee of the College of American Pathologists. The role of the autopsy in medical malpractice cases, I: a review of 99 appeals court decisions. Arch Pathol Lab Med. 2002;126(9):1023–31.
27. Casali MB, Mobilia F, Del Sordo S, Blandino A, Genovese U. The medical malpractice in Milan-Italy. A retrospective survey on 14 years of judicial autopsies. Forensic Sci Int. 2014;242:38–43.
28. Bove KE, Iery C, Autopsy Committee of the College of American Pathologists. The role of the autopsy in medical malpractice cases, II: controversy related to autopsy performance and reporting. Arch Pathol Lab Med. 2002;126(9):1032–5.
29. Langlois NE. The use of histology in 638 coronial post-mortem examinations of adults: an audit. Med Sci Law. 2006;46(4):310–20.

30. Scientific Working Group for Medicolegal Death Investigation. Regional medicolegal autopsy and death investigation centers: construction, staffing, and costs. 17 Sept 2013. https://swgmdi.org/images/si6.facilityconstruction.published.9-17-13.pdf. Accessed 21 Apr 2018.
31. Seelye KQ. Opioid deaths taking a toll on medical examiners' offices. The Seattle times October 7 2017. https://www.seattletimes.com/nation-world/opioid-deaths-taking-a-toll-on-medical-examiners-offices/. Accessed 21 Apr 2018.
32. Valaske MJ. Loss control/risk management. A survey of the contribution of autopsy examination. Arch Pathol Lab Med. 1984;108(6):462–8.

Part III

Autopsy Practice in the Modern Era

Essential Techniques in Certain Decedent Populations

5

Kim A. Collins

Introduction

The autopsy has been used in science and medicine since 300 BCE [1]. However, over the last few decades, the value of the autopsy has increased due to advances in and utilization of ancillary techniques [2]. Not every case will use every or even a majority of these techniques, but based on the decedent, certain ancillary studies should be undertaken to allow accurate certification of the cause and manner of death, as well as to identify any underlying congenital, hereditary, or contributory conditions or diseases. As science and medicine advance, epidemiologists have studied trends in worldwide populations to identify and prevent diseases. The autopsy is the greatest tool for public health. No matter how extensive and "cutting edge" clinical diagnostic modalities become, the autopsy ("to see for oneself") gives true final pathologic diagnoses and accurate causes of death. It expands and enhances data on every disease, inherent and acquired, in all people. It also identifies populations at risk so that diseases can be prevented. The autopsy identifies new diseases and different subsets of society particularly vulnerable to these new diseases. Answers to questions from all branches of medicine can be found in the autopsy.

As societies around the world change and develop, social norms, fads, dangers, and behavioral trends emerge. The autopsy often reflects these changes via pathologic diagnoses, causes of death, incidental findings, and manners of death. A routine autopsy is not actually routine. The autopsy pathologist must always strive to correlate the history with the autopsy findings and, if no known correlation exists, find it. New findings and new diagnoses will be overlooked if each decedent is examined in exactly the same way and by the same methods as in the preceding

K. A. Collins
Newberry Pathology Associates, Newberry, SC, USA

Sharing Hope South Carolina, Charleston, SC, USA

J. E. Hooper, A. K. Williamson (eds.), *Autopsy in the 21st Century*,
https://doi.org/10.1007/978-3-319-98373-8_5

hundreds of years. This chapter will discuss postmortem techniques and studies that have proven useful in autopsy pathology. It will also discuss special patient populations that present unique challenges to the autopsy pathologist. In order to see for oneself, we need to know what we are looking at and what we should be looking for.

Basic Science

Postmortem Chemistry

Biochemical analyses of postmortem specimens and proper interpretation of the results can be extremely beneficial to the pathologist. Often when gross and microscopic autopsy findings are "negative," chemistry can provide answers. A brief overview of postmortem chemistry is needed to better approach certain cases [3–14].

Vitreous humor is the best specimen for analyzing concentrations of electrolytes, glucose, and ketones [2–4, 14]. Other low-molecular-weight, nonprotein-bound solutes such as ethanol can also be measured. Vitreous should be collected from the globe using a sterile syringe (usually 10 mL) and needle (18–20 gauge) with the needle inserted at the lateral canthus and directed to the center of the globe [2]. The vitreous should be withdrawn slowly and placed into a small, sterile, red-top vacutainer. Vitreous is a viscous, clear, colorless fluid. If the specimen is contaminated with retinal cells, the results will not be reliable. When interpreting vitreous chemistry results, it is important to understand that some postmortem vitreous values do not reflect premortem blood values of a given analyte. For instance, after death, potassium quickly leaks from the retina resulting in elevated levels in the vitreous. On the other hand, vitreous glucose concentrations fall rapidly after death. The College of American Pathologists published a useful reference table for vitreous chemistry results and their correlation with some entities likely to be encountered in hospitalized patients [2–14]. A basic metabolic panel to include these tests can be performed on postmortem vitreous by a hospital's chemistry laboratory.

Toxicology

Toxicology can be useful in non-forensic deaths as well as forensic cases, and hospital autopsists may be called upon to assist local medical examiner offices with collecting toxicology specimens, especially considering the growing opioid epidemic (see Chaps. 4 and 7 in this book for more details). Clinicians may be concerned about the blood concentration of a drug in the setting of liver or kidney disease or in neonates with seizures with possible transplacental drug overdose, as examples. The best specimen for a toxicology screen is urine (approximately 30–50 mL) collected in a sterile container. For confirmation and quantitation, the best specimen is femoral venous blood placed in a gray-top vacutainer which contains the preservative sodium fluoride [2]. The preservative must be thoroughly mixed with the blood by gently rolling and inverting the vacutainer. Gastric contents should be examined for pills or pill fragments, quantitated, and a portion (50 mL) either analyzed or saved frozen in a sterile container. The liver, brain, and skeletal muscle are also good specimens to save (35–50 g of each), frozen if needed. Meconium (the first feces in a newborn) is an excellent specimen for toxicology. The thick, viscous meconium can be placed in a sterile red-top tube. The aforementioned specimens can be stored for many years at 4–6 °C.

Table 5.1 Dictionary of basic terms for special decedent populations

Term	Definition
Infectious diseases	
Bacteremia	The presence of bacteria in the bloodstream
Hypotension	Low blood pressure, usually less than 90/60 mmHg
Sepsis	Systemic response to bacterial, viral, fungal, or parasitic infection
Septic shock	Clinical syndrome of sepsis with critical reduction in tissue perfusion
SIRS	Response to infection, inflammation, and/or insult to the body
Toxic shock syndrome	Special type of shock caused by bacterial toxins
DIC	Systemic activation of blood coagulation resulting in excessive bleeding
Perinatal and infant decedents	
Embryo	Product of conception to the end of 8 weeks gestation
Fetus	Product of conception from 9 weeks gestation to birth
Neonate	A child from the time of birth to 1 month of age
Infant	A child between 1 and 12 months of age
Congenital	A genetic or non-genetic condition present in an individual at birth
Elder decedents	
Elder	Someone who is at least 60 years of age
Biologic aging	Changes of organs and tissues with advancing age
Atrophy	Wasting due to degeneration of cells and tissues
Decubitus ulcer	Damage to skin and underlying tissue due to prolonged pressure
Eating disorders	
Adiposity	The amount of body fat can be expressed as a percentage of body mass
Obesity	Excessive accumulation and storage of fat in the body (BMI at least 30)
BMI	Body mass index, mass in kilograms divided by length in meters squared
Anorexia nervosa	Eating disorder characterized by distorted body image and intentional weight loss
Bulimia nervosa	Eating disorder characterized by periods of binging followed by purging
Anabolic steroid	Steroidal androgen that promotes growth of skeletal muscle and male sexual traits

Infectious Diseases

Table 5.1 provides a dictionary of basic terms to be used in this section as well as several following sections of this chapter. Please also refer to Table 5.1 for definitions of key terms later in the text.

Infectious diseases result in many deaths in all age groups, and autopsy findings can be subtle. Some diseases such as bacterial pneumonia may be obvious upon gross examination, whereas others such as influenza provide no anatomic clues of their presence. Some basic definitions relating to postmortem evaluation of clinically suspected infections are important to bear in mind when reviewing clinical records and correlating pathology with clinical history in cases of suspected infectious deaths.

Sepsis and Sepsis Syndromes

Sepsis is a life-threatening organ dysfunction caused by a dysregulated host response to an infection [15–23]. Septic shock is a critical reduction in tissue perfusion and abnormalities of cellular metabolism due to the infection, and it involves persistent hypotension and an elevated serum lactate level [19, 20]. The systemic inflammatory response syndrome (SIRS) is a specifically defined response and has four criteria [19, 20, 22]:

- Fever of more than 38 °C (100.4 °F) or hypothermia less than 36 °C (96.8 °F)
- Tachycardia (heart rate of more than 90 beats per minute)
- Tachypnea (respiratory rate of more than 20 breaths per minute) or hyperventilation with arterial carbon dioxide tension (PaCO2) of less than 32 mmHg
- Abnormal white blood cell count (>12,000/μL or < 4000/μL) or presence of immature neutrophils (>10% immature [band] forms)

SIRS has been used to identify early sepsis, but the criteria lack sensitivity and specificity for identifying increased mortality risk [19, 20, 22]. The sequential organ failure assessment (SOFA) scoring system is another method of predicting mortality in such situations and involves assessment of three criteria: respiratory rate ≥ 22 breaths per minute, change in mental status, and systolic blood pressure ≤ 100 mmHg [18].

Another dire consequence of systemic infection is disseminated intravascular coagulation (DIC), also known as consumptive coagulopathy. Eventually, the activation of coagulation depletes the coagulation proteins and platelets resulting in excessive bleeding. At autopsy, hemorrhage can be seen in the skin, mucocutaneous tissues, serosal membranes, and various organs. Platelet and fibrin thrombi can be histologically identified, especially in the renal glomeruli and pulmonary alveolar capillaries.

Two purported laboratory markers consistent with sepsis include C-reactive protein (CRP), a protein produced in the liver in response to inflammation, and procalcitonin, the precursor, or prohormone, to calcitonin which is secreted in response to inflammatory stimulation.

Utility of Postmortem Cultures

When bacteremia or sepsis is suspected, it is important to perform the autopsy as soon as possible (ideally within 18–24 h of death) and be prepared to take various cultures and specimens for microbiology/virology testing [24–28]. If medical records are available, a thorough review is strongly encouraged before beginning the autopsy, noting relevant vital signs and laboratory results, including antemortem microbiology findings.

The postmortem evaluation of a patient assumed to be infected is twofold. First, the presence and location of an infection must be determined, and second, the likelihood of morbidity and mortality from sepsis must be assessed. Clinicians have attempted to develop various criteria and scores to help them evaluate the severity of a patient's status [17–19, 21, 23]. The listed terminologies often overlap in individual cases but are also not absolute in every case. For example, not all infections result in SIRS, and not all cases of SIRS are secondary to infection. However, an infection plus SIRS is associated with organ dysfunction and substantial mortality in 5–16% of cases [22]. An infection in one location may stay localized, but toxins (such as in TSS) and/or an activated immune system can cause damage at distant sites. The SOFA scoring system is used to assess the severity of organ dysfunction and thus morbidity [18]. The predictive validity of the SOFA score for mortality has been reported to be superior to that of the SIRS criteria. Unfortunately, the applications of these criteria and scores vary between hospitals and between clinicians.

For the autopsy pathologist, it is important to know the clinical status of the patient. The clinical history, including microbiology culture results or presence of shock or organ dysfunction, can be correlated to the autopsy findings [2, 24–30]. Infections are among the 15 leading causes of death in the United States. Therefore, a thorough understanding of the different clinical pictures of sepsis is important in the interpretation of gross and microscopic autopsy findings as well as interpreting postmortem ancillary studies.

Performance of Postmortem Cultures

Controversy exists over the performance of postmortem microbiology cultures because there is confusion over their interpretation [2, 25–28]. Many studies have cited the lack of agreement between premortem and postmortem blood cultures [25]. There are several possible reasons for this which can be divided into two main categories: postmortem bacterial transmigration and iatrogenic contamination. Indigenous visceral microbial flora can transmigrate after death and spread throughout the body. To lessen this postmortem effect, the body should be cooled promptly after death, and body mobilization should be limited, as well. The autopsy should be performed as soon as reasonably possible, best within 15 h postmortem. To limit iatrogenic contamination, attention must be paid to using sterile technique when procuring blood, body fluid, exudate, or tissue for microbiology culture.

Growth of a single commonly recognized pathogen can usually be considered a true indicator of antemortem infection, whereas growth of multiple organisms and/or growth of a typical contaminant can usually be considered postmortem artifact due to transmigration and/or iatrogenic contamination (Table 5.2). Correlation of postmortem microbiology cultures with microscopic autopsy findings is of great value, as is corroborating histologic inflammation in a site from which cultures were taken.

So why perform postmortem blood or tissue cultures? Several good reasons exist despite the aforementioned controversy. First, a positive culture can determine the cause of death. Secondly, the autopsy pathologist can identify the agent as the cause of a previously undiagnosed infection even if that infection is not the proximate cause of death. Thirdly, postmortem cultures can confirm the premortem diagnosis and be of value in evaluating clinical assessment and response to antimicrobial treatment. Finally, public health benefits when epidemics and evolving antimicrobial resistance cannot be over emphasized.

Culture Techniques for Microbiology and Virology

When taking blood for culture, sterile technique must be used. If it can be performed safely, one preferred method is to sear the right cardiac atrium with a heated spatula or wide blade before inserting the sterile needle with syringe [2, 14, 24–28]. Another method is to flood the area with iodine and then insert the needle with syringe. Using a sterile needle and sterile syringe, withdraw 20–30 ml of blood for

Table 5.2 Common blood pathogens and blood contaminants

Common blood pathogens	Common blood contaminants
Staphylococcus aureus	Coagulase-negative staphylococci
Streptococcus pneumoniae *Streptococcus pyogenes* *Streptococcus agalactiae*	*Streptococcus viridans*
No common parallel pathogen	*Propionibacterium acnes*
No common parallel pathogen	Corynebacterium
Enterobacteriaceae	Mixed intestinal flora
Bacillus anthracis	Bacillus (other species)
Neisseria gonorrhoeae, meningitidis	*Neisseria subflava,* other species
Listeria monocytogenes	No parallel contaminant
Bacteroides fragilis	Mixed intestinal flora
Pseudomonas aeruginosa	No common parallel gram-negative contaminants
Haemophilus influenzae	
Escherichia coli	
Candida albicans	No common contaminants, though fungi often present in autopsy environment
Cryptococcus neoformans	

the aerobic and anaerobic culture/broth bottles. The rubber top of the bottle (where the needle is to be inserted) should be sterilized by iodine followed by isopropyl alcohol or sterilized by isopropyl alcohol alone. The inoculated bottle should be promptly transported to the microbiology laboratory.

Any organ or tissue can be cultured by the use of a culturette or a sterile biopsy [2, 14, 24]. The culturette can detect aerobic organisms and fungi. For organ/tissue biopsy, the surface of the organ is seared or flooded with iodine, as above, and a sterile blade is used to cut out a section of the tissue. Sterile aerobic and anaerobic transport media should be used. To maintain the anaerobic environment, make sure that the tissue is pressed into and covered by the solid media. Tissues can also be analyzed for viruses.

Mycobacteria can be detected from various specimens including blood, tissue, and feces. Mycobacterium can grow out of conventional blood culture media, but Middlebrook broth is recommended. The laboratory must be informed that mycobacterium is a consideration because laboratory smears, special stains, and special growth media will need to be used.

Rapid tests, usually utilizing molecular techniques such as polymerase chain reaction (PCR), are available for several viruses including respiratory and gastrointestinal viruses [31]. Blood procured and placed into a serum separator vacutainer can be analyzed for viral antibodies. Tissues for culture can be procured using sterile technique as described above, placed into viral media such as Hanks solution, and immediately transported on ice to the laboratory. Paraffin-embedded tissues can also be analyzed for viruses using immunohistochemistry and molecular diagnostic assays [30, 32–34]. Sometimes tissues will need to be sent to a reference laboratory for analysis. These can be paraffin-embedded formalin-fixed or fresh tissues [2, 24, 30, 34].

Fresh tissue samples for respiratory viruses can be procured by sterile technique, as above, and placed in a sterile container with a small amount of sterile saline. If they are to be shipped to a reference laboratory, the samples may need to be frozen. The following samples should be taken: bilateral lung hila, epiglottis, larynx, bilateral proximal and distal bronchi, and representative sections of bilateral lung parenchyma. Other organs and tissues may likewise be procured by sterile technique and frozen. Fecal specimens (10–20 ml) for viruses can also be collected in a sterile container and frozen for shipment to a reference laboratory. Some hospital laboratories have rapid viral enteritis tests and can microscopically examine for other agents of gastrointestinal infectious disease, such as parasites [31].

Perinatal and Infant Decedents

Important Procedures for Perinatal and Infant Decedents

Records Medical records of both the mother and the deceased child are extremely important to review before starting the autopsy. These include prenatal records, delivery records, and pediatric records as well as any required state genetic testing results.

Growth Measurements External measurements should be taken of all decedents 5 years of age and under. These include head circumference (occipital-frontal circumference), chest circumference (at the nipple line), abdominal circumference (at the umbilicus), crown-rump length (top of head to bottom of buttocks), crown-heel length (top of head to bottom of heel), and foot length (back of heel to end of great toe). These measurements should be compared to expected values for the age of the child. Charts for prematurely born children are available. See the following section on body mass index (BMI).

The best way to obtain accurate circumference measurements is to wrap a string around the body part (e.g., head) and then place the string along a ruler to obtain the circumference length.

Radiographs Full-body radiographs should be performed, and a skeletal survey including AP views of the skull, thorax, abdomen, individual limbs, hands, and feet and lateral views of the skull and thorax is highly recommended beyond the fetal age. Review by a pediatric radiologist can be very instrumental in assessing genetic defects, nutritional status, and birth or subsequent trauma. Previous radiographs should be obtained and reviewed for comparison, when possible.

Placenta In cases of perinatal or neonatal death, the placenta provides "the answer" in over one-third of the cases. The placental disc should be weighed without the umbilical cord and membranes. The membranes should be thoroughly examined for color and transparency. The umbilical cord length and diameter should be recorded and any unusual coiling noted. The site of cord insertion should be recorded. There is disagreement as to whether the placenta should be refrigerated (not frozen), unfixed, or fixed in 10% formalin. If refrigerated, the placenta can be stored at 4 °C for 3–7 days without loss of histologic integrity. The placenta ideally should be placed in a large, flat container so as not to distort its shape. The placenta should not be frozen because freezing results in lysis of red blood cells and marked distortion of histology. Keeping the placenta fresh (unfixed) allows for tissue procurement and the use of certain ancillary studies, such as bacterial and viral cultures, DNA and cytogenetic studies, metabolic studies, electron microscopy, and infusion studies. Tissue for bacterial and viral cultures may be taken in a sterile fashion from the subamniotic chorionic plate. The membranes also may be swabbed with a culturette for bacterial cultures. Sections of the fetal aspect of the placental disc can also be obtained for cytogenetic studies. If the placenta has already been discarded, or if it has been examined at another institution, the placental slides and accompanying pathology report should be reviewed by the autopsist.

For microscopic examination of placentas, the following sections should be submitted: (1) at least two full-thickness sections of the placental disc, (2) umbilical cord cross-sections from the fetal and placental ends, and (3) two sections of the placental membrane roll.

Microbiology Cultures If sufficient blood is not available due to the age (size) of the child, the spleen can be cultured. Lung cultures can be very valuable in this age group and should be taken. Sections of tissue, such as the liver and lung, or serum for viruses can be taken if a virus is suspected or for future analysis. Culture results can be correlated with histological findings as well as immunohistochemistry. See discussion of cultures.

Evisceration Technique In older children and adults, many pathologists use the Virchow method (organ by organ removal) of evisceration. However, in the perinatal and young pediatric age groups, when abnormal anatomical arrangements and/or vascular connections may not be immediately apparent, the en bloc or Letulle (also more recently referred to as Rokitansky) approach is advised so that anatomic relationships remain intact for evaluation. Remove the neck, thorax, abdominal, and pelvic block and begin the examination and dissection from the posterior aspect. The esophagus should be opened along its length to identify any tracheoesophageal fistula, before being taken down to the abdominal block. The heart-lung vascular connections should be carefully examined.

Fetal Brain Removal The fetal and often neonatal brain is very soft due to increased water content and can prove difficult to remove without damaging important landmarks and architecture. To avoid too many artifacts, cut open the fontanelles and sutures with scissors, cut the brain attachments, and gently remove the brain. In cases of very early gestation or maceration, removing the brain under water can best preserve its architecture.

Organ Weights In fetal, perinatal, and pediatric cases, especially 13 years of age and younger, it is important to compare the decedent's organ weights to expected weights for similar decedents. The expected weight is best based on the child's body (or crown-heel for fetuses) length. Expected body measurement and organ weight charts for prematurely born infants are available and are especially important for meaningful evaluation of premature babies and young children.

Genetic/Chromosomal Abnormalities and Inborn Errors of Metabolism Blood in an EDTA tube or blood as a spot on filter paper can be analyzed for numerous inborn errors of metabolism. Sections of the skin, fascia lata, and Achilles' tendon may be taken for fibroblast culture and cytogenetics and enzyme deficiencies. Skin sections (1 cm^3), and one or two entire Achilles' tendons, and fascia lata, taken using sterile technique, should be placed in transport media such as Hank's solution, and immediately transported on ice to the laboratory. Molecular pathology can be performed on paraffin-embedded sections using fluorescent in situ hybridization (FISH) or polymerase chain reaction (PCR) methodologies.

Many cardiac channelopathies can be detected in postmortem specimens. Blood, 5–10 mL, collected in an EDTA purple-top vacutainer is the specimen of choice. Other possible specimens include at least 5 g of fresh heart, liver, or spleen. The fresh tissues should then be frozen. Contact the reference laboratory for more specific instructions.

Postmortem Chemistry Vitreous should be procured for chemical analysis as described above. In children under 5 years of age, procurement of vitreous is usually performed at the end of the autopsy. This is because if any head pathology is identified, the eyes may need to be examined without any artifact of vitreous withdrawal.

Examination of the Elder Patient

In 2012, 809 million people, or 11% of the world's population, were over age 60. By 2050, about two billion people are expected to be over age 60, which will represent nearly 22% of the world's population at that time [35]. Life expectancy for the US population in 2016 was 78.6 years (males = 76.1 years, females = 81.1 years) [35]. Almost 40% of elders as defined above are obese, putting them at risk for diseases such as systemic hypertension, diabetes mellitus, coronary atherosclerosis, cerebral infarction, renal disease, respiratory diseases, decreased mobility, osteoarthritis, and cancer [35–39].

It is therefore not surprising that the top ten causes of death in this age group are [35]:

1. Heart disease
2. Malignant neoplasm
3. Chronic lower respiratory disease
4. Cerebrovascular disease
5. Alzheimer disease
6. Diabetes mellitus
7. Unintentional injury
8. Pneumonia and influenza
9. Nephritis, nephrotic syndrome, and nephrosis
10. Septicemia

As with children, specific approaches need to be taken when examining the elder decedent. With age, changes in the body make a person more prone to or at risk for various diseases and trauma.

Pathophysiology of Aging

A description by organ system of changes related to biologic aging, as well as to underlying pathologies that tend to be more prevalent with aging, follows and is summarized in Table 5.3 [36, 41, 42].

Table 5.3 The pathophysiology of aging and associated autopsy findings

Body systems	Effects of aging	Autopsy finding
Integumentary system	Thinning skin, fragile blood vessels, immobility, poor blood flow	Ecchymoses, decubitus ulcers, stigmata of diabetes
Musculoskeletal system	Decreased bone mass, Less vitamin D production, muscle mass decreased	Osteopenia, osteoporosis, fractures, muscle atrophy
Cardiovascular system	High cholesterol, high blood pressure	CAD, myocardial infarction, thrombosis, myocardial interstitial fibrosis
Respiratory system	Difficulty breathing, less ability to expand lungs and chest	Pneumonia, emphysema
Gastrointestinal system	Dry mouth, decreased gag reflex, decreased gastric secretions, slow digestion	Periodontal disease, aspiration, fecal impaction
Genitourinary system	Decreased blood flow to kidneys (vascular disease)	Kidney atrophy, glomerulosclerosis, arteriosclerosis
Hepatobiliary system	Decreased blood flow to liver	Liver atrophy, Glycogenated hepatocyte nuclei
Central nervous system	Trouble with walking and balance, greater fall risk, loss of memory	Brain atrophy, atherosclerosis, increased neurofibrillary tangles, subdural hemorrhage

Integumentary System The skin becomes thin with decreased elasticity, and often effects of long-term sun exposure are present, as well. The epidermis can be easily separated from the underlying dermis with minimal trauma due to flattened dermal-epidermal junctions and decreased interdigitations. The skeletal muscle is atrophied, and subcutaneous adipose tissue is overall decreased. The blood vessels can become fragile and decreased in number. Resultant senile purpura and senile ecchymosis, especially over the extensor surfaces and over bony prominences, are seen. Also, anticoagulant medications and drug-induced thrombocytopenias can result in easy bruisability. Underlying peripheral vascular disease and/or diabetes mellitus puts the elder at risk for poor wound healing, pressure ulcers, and infections. Decreased hair over the lower legs and other cutaneous signs of vascular stasis is also indicative of peripheral vascular disease.

A decubitus ulcer, also termed a pressure ulcer, is usually due to immobility, and the tissue breakdown is enhanced by urinary and/or fecal incontinence, malnutrition, a decrease in overall body fat including subcutaneous adipose tissue, muscular atrophy due to aging, decreased immunity, aforementioned skin fragility, vascular insufficiency due to atherosclerosis and/or diabetes mellitus, and generally delayed wound healing. Pressure sores can be divided into four stages [42]:

- Stage 1 Non-blanchable erythema of intact skin
- Changes in sensation, temperature, or firmness may precede visual changes.
- Stage 2 Partial-thickness skin loss with exposed dermis

- Partial-thickness loss of the skin with exposed dermis. The wound bed is viable, pink or red, and moist and may also present as an intact or ruptured serum-filled blister. These injuries commonly result from adverse microclimate and shearing forces, particularly over the pelvis and heels. This stage should not be used to describe moisture-associated skin damage (MASD) including incontinence-associated dermatitis (IAD), intertriginous dermatitis (ITD), medical adhesive-related skin injury (MARSI), or traumatic wounds (skin tears, burns, abrasions).
- Stage 3 Full-thickness skin loss
- Subcutaneous adipose tissue may be visible in the bottom of the wound, and the ulcer may include granulation tissue and epibole (rolled wound edges), but the underlying fibrous tissue, muscle, or bone are not visible. Sloughing and/or eschar may be present and undermining and tunneling may occur. If slough or eschar obscures the extent of tissue loss this is an unstageable pressure injury.
- Stage 4 Full-thickness skin and tissue loss
- Exposed or directly palpable fascia, muscle, tendon, ligament, cartilage, or bone in the ulcer. Slough and/or eschar may be visible. Epibole, undermining, and/or tunneling often also occur [42].

Musculoskeletal System With age, there is often decreased bone mass and less vitamin D production, with consequent osteoporosis and osteopenia, respectively, as well as decreased flexibility. These changes can result in fractures due to falls and sternal and rib fractures during cardiopulmonary resuscitation. Fractures seen in accidental trauma occur most often in the femoral neck, vertebrae, proximal humerus, and ribs. Muscle mass is decreased with age but can also be due to wasting secondary to immobility, chronic disease, malabsorption, dysphagia, and lack of proper caloric intake and nutrition [36, 37, 41].

Cardiovascular System With age comes increased incidence of or risk for atherosclerosis, valve stenosis, and cardiovascular effects of long-term systemic hypertension. The cardiac output is also decreased. Long-term systemic hypertension can lead to myocyte hypertrophy and replacement fibrosis. The elder may develop acquired thrombotic tendencies. Decreased peripheral vasoconstriction and vasodilation, often coupled with decreased sweat response in the skin, can lead to hypothermia and hyperthermia, as well.

Respiratory System The lungs have decreased elastic recoil, decreased pulmonary reserve, and overall decreased lung mechanics with decreased chest compliance and strength of respiratory muscles. Therefore, elders are prone to pneumonia. Underlying pulmonary emphysema is not uncommon in this population, as well.

Gastrointestinal System Elders often have dry mouth, or xerostomia, secondary to aging or to certain medications. Xerostomia can result in periodontal disease, cavities, and difficulty swallowing. Decreased gag reflex can also cause dysphagia and lead to aspiration. The senses of taste and smell are decreased. Medications can also alter the sense of taste. Appetite decreases with aging as does the sense of thirst. Elders have slower gastrointestinal peristalsis which can lead to fecal impaction. Decreased gastric secretions and intestinal enzymes can result in malabsorption. Colonic diverticular disease and diverticulitis are also prevalent in this population.

Genitourinary System The decreased cardiac output and atherosclerosis result in decreased blood flow to the kidneys. The kidneys have a decreased number of nephrons, decreased glomerular filtration rate, impaired water absorption, decreased urine concentration ability, and decreased creatinine clearance [36, 37, 41]. In women, decreased estrogens lead to vaginal atrophy. Increased vaginal pH can promote infections. The pelvic wall structures weaken and can result in a cystocele or uterine prolapse.

Hepatobiliary System The liver volume is decreased, at least partly due to decreased blood flow to the liver. Microscopically, hepatocytes often have glycogenated nuclei, not only in those individuals with diabetes mellitus but also as a marker of hepatocyte senescence in most aging individuals. Hepatocytes also have lipofuscin accumulation which can interfere with cellular pathways. Decreased hepatic metabolism, especially decrease in the P450 enzyme activity, can interfere with drug metabolism. Liver regeneration capacity is also decreased [43].

Central Nervous System The elder brain is atrophied with decreased weight. The cerebral ventricles can be enlarged due to the atrophy of the surrounding parenchyma. An enlarged subdural space puts the elder at risk for subdural hemorrhage secondary to a fall. The brain has decreased blood flow and decreased neurotransmitters. It is not uncommon to see atherosclerosis of the basilar artery and circle of Willis, meningeal edema, remote infarctions, and lacunar infarctions in the basal ganglia. Age-related increase in neurofibrillary tangles can be seen, including in the parahippocampal gyrus and amygdala. Elders can have impaired gait, decreased proprioception, and slower reaction times, putting them at risk for falls and resultant intracranial injury [36].

Performing the Elder Autopsy

Body Measurements

Weigh the body unclothed and measure body length [36–39, 41]. Find out if the weight has changed dramatically over the past 12 months or if there has been a noticeable trend (especially weight loss) over the past few years. It is important to calculate a body mass index (BMI), but pathologists must also understand that a loss of weight can also accompany other pathologies such as dementia.

Radiographs

Full-body radiographs can be considered if there is any history of or findings suspicious for trauma or neglect. Radiographs will detect fractures (acute, healing, and possibly remote), reveal abnormal mineralization, and suggest osteomyelitis (especially beneath pressure ulcers).

Toxicology

The vitreous should be analyzed for electrolytes, glucose, and ketones [2, 4, 14]. Dehydration, renal failure, diabetes mellitus, and diabetic ketoacidosis are some entities that may be discovered. An elder's medication level may be elevated due to decreased metabolism and clearance. The level may be low if the medications have not been taken or administered.

Autopsy Procedures

Below are a few remarks or "tips" about autopsy procedures in the elderly. After a thorough external and internal examination possibly including radiographs, the pathologist may want to alter what would ordinarily be the "routine" autopsy procedure.

- Measure the thickness of the abdominal panniculus to correlate with weight in cases of cachexia, malnutrition, or an otherwise underweight elder.
- Perform and document an oral examination.
- If trauma is identified grossly or radiographically, it is worthwhile to do a posterior Y incision exposing the back and buttocks to identify any occult subcutaneous or muscular injury.
- Native coronary arteries and any bypass grafts should be dissected, examined, and submitted for histology.
- If the small and large bowels are not routinely opened, they should be in elder cases. Document and appropriately evaluate the consistency of fecal material, volume of bowel contents including feces in cases of suspected neglect, and any pathology such as tumors or diverticuli.
- If the decedent has pressure sores, the ulcer can be cultured and sectioned for histology, especially the bone to evaluate for underlying osteomyelitis.
- Full neuropathologic examination with relevant sections should be performed in cases of suspected or known dementia.

The elder autopsy is often complicated by diseases in multiple organ systems which can confuse the diagnostic picture. Remember that many elders will die with their diseases and not necessarily of their diseases. Take time to differentiate disease that is relevant from disease that is irrelevant to the cause of death [36, 40].

Autopsy of Individuals with Eating Disorders

Deaths can result from eating disorders including obesity, anorexia nervosa, and bulimia nervosa with or without anorexia nervosa. Death due to the use of supplements and steroids can also fall into this category.

Obesity

Worldwide obesity has nearly tripled since 1975 [44–62]. In fact, in 2016 almost two billion adults worldwide age 18 years and older were overweight, and over 650 million were diagnosed as obese. Also, in 2016, 41 million children under the age of 5 years fell into the categories of overweight or obese. From 5 to 9 years of age, over 340 million children were overweight or obese [49–52]. In the United States in 2016, almost 40% of adults were considered obese [45–47]. Between the ages of 2 and 19 years, 18.5% of children were obese [45–47, 50–55].

Overweight and obese conditions are defined as an abnormal or excessive fat accumulation, respectively, that may impair health [48, 49]. Since these definitions are subjective, methods have been devised to allow physicians and the public to better categorize disorders of fat accumulation. BMI, body mass index, is an anthropometric index of weight and height that is defined as body mass in kilograms divided by the height in meters squared [54]. BMI is a screening tool to classify adiposity. In other words, BMI assists the clinician and pathologist in categorizing a patient as being of normal weight, underweight, overweight, or obese. The BMI does have its limitations as it uses height and weight and does not directly measure body adiposity. More definitive measures of body fat are skinfold thickness, bioelectrical impedance analysis, and dual energy X-ray absorptiometry (considered the gold standard).

Because adiposity varies with age and gender, the BMI changes substantially between the age of 2 years up to 20 years [50–56]. Therefore, BMI-for-age charting based on gender should be used. BMI-for-age is better than the standard pediatric weight-height charts in assessing underweight and overweight children as it takes into account age-related changes that occur in early childhood and in puberty. BMI in children correlates with cardiovascular disease, systemic hypertension, hyperlipidemia, and hyperinsulinemia later in life. BMI under the age of 2 years has a weak association with adiposity and future obesity and, therefore, is not used in this age group.

Obesity is associated with comorbidities and a decreased life expectancy [57–62]. The life expectancy is decreased by 6 years in obese men and by 7 years in obese females. Obese individuals are more likely to die before the age of 70 years.

The top four causes of death in obese individuals are malignancy, infection, heart disease, and pulmonary thromboembolus.

Obese individuals should be weighed and measured (unclothed). The BMI can then be calculated. Make sure that when the body length is measured, that the tape measure is flat on the table and not over the decedent's protuberant abdomen, creating a false increase in length. Radiographs can be helpful to assess degenerative changes to the bones and joints, even in obese children. The CDC BMI-for-age growth charts show BMI as a percentile ranking for children 2–19 years of age. BMI can be calculated, but the distribution of fat is also of concern since intra-abdominal (visceral) fat is associated with cardiovascular disease. BMI is a screening evaluation, and, in some circumstances such as users of anabolic androgenic steroids (discussed later in this chapter), a high BMI does not correlate with adiposity.

Effects of Obesity

Organs most often adversely affected by obesity are the heart, liver, and kidneys [58]. The heart is usually increased in weight secondary to increased blood volume and systemic hypertension, as well as fat deposition externally and within the myocytes. In men, the enlarged heart often shows an increase in the left ventricular thickness, whereas in women the heart weight is increased with an increase in both the left and right ventricular thicknesses [58]. Cardiac uptake and oxidation of fats are not balanced, and the heart accumulates lipid leading to lipotoxicity. The fat deposits can directly alter cellular structures, are toxic to myocytes, and alter systolic and diastolic function. Obesity can also be associated with accelerated atherosclerosis. The liver is often enlarged with steatosis accompanied by ballooning and degenerating hepatocytes and acute inflammation. Nonalcoholic fatty liver disease and nonalcoholic steatohepatitis can occur secondary to obesity. Obese individuals and those with type II diabetes mellitus (DM) commonly have glycogen accumulation in the hepatic nuclei. Kidneys can be scarred secondary to glomerulosclerosis, arteriolosclerosis, and arteriosclerosis resulting in chronic renal failure. For some reason, in men with an elevated BMI, the thyroid gland is often increased in weight [58].

Obese individuals can develop type II diabetes mellitus (DM) due to a progressive defect in insulin secretion coupled with a progressive rise in insulin resistance [62]. Obese individuals with type II DM are at risk for hyperglycemic hyperosmolar nonketotic sudden death, evidenced by elevated glucose but absence of ketones or ketone bodies in the vitreous.

Anorexia Nervosa

Anorexia nervosa (AN) is a psychological eating disorder characterized by a distorted body image and intentional weight loss [63–70]. Individuals with AN have an obsessive fear of weight gain, a distorted body image, refuse to eat to maintain a healthy body weight, and deny the serious consequences of such behavior. Most patients are women, and the average age of onset is 17 years. In the United States, 1–3% of women and 0.5% of men will experience AN during their lifetime [63–70]. Left untreated, 20–50% with AN will die. If treated, 15% will still likely die from complications of the disorder. One in five AN deaths is due to suicide. The anorexic decedent is markedly underweight with a BMI usually under 17.5. The decrease in body adipose tissue and muscle atrophy are apparent at autopsy. Vitreous chemistry may be positive for ketones as the body switches from carbohydrate to lipid energy sources [4]. If vomiting is induced, vitreous chloride will be decreased, as well. Some anorexic individuals abuse laxatives resulting in a low potassium level.

These individuals often have gastrointestinal disturbances including delayed motility and gastric dilatation as well as gastric smooth muscle atrophy. An acute gastric dilatation can result in gastric necrosis and perforation. Delayed gastric emptying followed by dilatation has also been reported to compress the inferior vena cava and superior mesenteric vein resulting in circulatory collapse.

One third of anorexic deaths are due to cardiac causes [65, 68]. Hypotension, bradycardia, repolarization abnormalities, arrhythmias, and prolonged QT interval are very common. Electrolyte imbalances, including low phosphorous and magnesium levels, can cause arrhythmias. Within the heart, one can see muscular atrophy including decreased left ventricular wall thickness resulting in mitral valve prolapse. Microscopically, myocytes are small, fragmented, display contraction bands, and have cytoplasmic accumulations of lipofuscin pigment.

Besides electrolyte abnormalities, severe muscle weakness, bulbar muscle dysfunction, and depressed diaphragmatic contractility can result in acute respiratory distress, aspiration, and sudden death. The immune system is markedly depressed and infections, sometimes fatal, are not uncommon. Death is usually caused by electrolyte imbalances and/or cardiac failure. Common findings at autopsy include low weight, lanugo hair, dry skin, acrocyanosis, and sometimes, hypercarotenemia (yellow skin). There may be osteoporosis, pressure ulcers, or malnutrition-induced hepatitis.

Bulimia Nervosa

Bulimia nervosa (BN) is an eating disorder characterized by periods of binging followed by purging [69, 71–73]. Clinically, it is defined as at least two binge eating episodes a week for a period of 3–6 months. BN is more common than AN but has a lower mortality of approximately 4%. Ten to fifteen percent of bulimics are males, and 85–95% are females [69, 71–73]. The age of onset is in the late teens. In the United States, 1.5% of people will suffer from BN. BN usually does not result in weight loss and can even cause weight gain. These individuals binge on an excessive amount of food, usually within a short time period, and, with a fear of gaining weight, then purge the consumed food. Purging can be accomplished by induced vomiting as well as the use of ipecac, laxatives, enemas, and diuretics.

Induced vomiting using one's hand can result in cuts, scars, and calluses on the dorsal middle phalanges (knuckles) from the teeth. The retching during vomiting can cause facial and ocular petechiae as small venules and capillaries rupture. Repeated vomiting erodes the enamel of the teeth leading to loss of enamel and tooth decay. Chronic gastric reflux with esophageal inflammation can also be seen. Repeated binging stretches the stomach and can actually damage the stomach lining resulting in tears and chemical peritonitis, or conversely, gastroparesis can result. The kidneys of individuals with longstanding bulimia nervosa can show chronic interstitial nephritis, proximal tubular swelling, and diffuse glomerulosclerosis. Death is usually the result of electrolyte imbalance.

Supplements and Anabolic Steroids

Many individuals take supplements in an attempt to change their body habitus, avoid medical procedures, substitute for traditional chemotherapy, treat medical conditions, and improve overall health. Unfortunately, too many of these supplements are not regulated, and the consumer may be unaware of the exact contents and/or side effects [74–79]. Besides often being ineffective, some contain harmful chemicals that can damage the body and even result in death [74, 76, 79]. For instance, supplements for weight loss may contain ephedrine, an arrhythmogenic agent. If a decedent is known to have taken supplements, the pathologist should obtain the exact supplement so that it can be used to interpret postmortem toxicology results.

Appearance and performance enhancing drugs (APEDs) are most often used by males to improve appearance by building muscle mass or to enhance athletic performance; however, they are also being used by females. Anabolic androgenic steroids are the best studied of the APEDs. These steroids are synthetic variations of the male sex hormone testosterone. People, men and women, take the steroid orally, inject them into veins or into the musculature, or apply them to the skin as creams, gels, or patches. Injection puts the user at risk for contracting and transmitting infections such as human immunodeficiency virus (HIV) and hepatitis C virus (HCV).

Steroids act on the brain and are addictive. They can produce mood swings including anger ("roid rage"), paranoia, and delusions. They do not trigger a rapid increase in the brain's dopamine, but, over time, they can affect the dopamine-serotonin-opiate sites and receptors [75, 77, 78]. At autopsy, the increase in muscle mass in both men and women is usually very obvious. The BMI of these individuals can be in the "obese" range because of the increased muscle mass. Below are other findings which may be seen at autopsy.

Integumentary System Men may show oily skin and hair and alopecia, as well as increased length and thickness of non-scalp hair, while women may show male pattern baldness or hirsutism and growth of facial hair.

Musculoskeletal System There is increased muscle mass and elevated BMI. Only in teens, stunted overall growth or height may be seen. There is often swelling of the hands and feet. Evidence of rhabdomyolysis, such as pigmented casts in the renal tubules, may be noted.

Cardiovascular System Cardiomegaly and left ventricular hypertrophy can occur. Accelerated atherosclerosis, coronary thrombosis, and patchy or interstitial myocardial fibrosis are often present.

Hepatobiliary System Cholestatic hepatitis may be found, as well as hepatic cysts and hepatocellular adenomas and carcinomas.

Genitourinary System Incidence of renal cell carcinoma may be increased, as well as prostatic hypertrophy and cancer in men. Spermatogenesis may be decreased. The clitoris may be enlarged in women, and there may be uterine and breast atrophy. Other microscopic findings in the kidney may include glomerulosclerosis, tubular atrophy or acute necrosis, and interstitial fibrosis.

The Present and the Future

Challenging postmortem cases are often those of sudden or unexpected deaths in which the routine autopsy is no longer the "routine." Cases with an uncommon cause of death, those which have nonspecific gross and microscopic findings, and cases involving unusual case histories can leave the pathologist perplexed and frustrated. Fortunately, advances have been made in several areas of laboratory medicine as well as non-pathology medicine, and many of these are applicable to the autopsy [80–82]. Also, a better understanding of complex pathophysiology such as infectious diseases and SIRS can help unravel what at first seems to be a web of unrelated signs, symptoms, and autopsy findings. Pathology and its many subspecialty branches are continuously evolving and advancing; autopsy pathology should change, as well.

In 1971, the Joint Commission on Accreditation of Hospitals dropped the hospital accreditation standard requiring a 20–25% autopsy rate for deaths occurring in the hospital [83–86]. In 1964, the US hospital autopsy rate was approximately 41%. By 2003, this rate had dropped to 11%, and by 2007 it was at 8.5% [85–95]. The effects of this drop on resident education, in particular pathology residents, are detailed in Chap. 6 of this book. Exposure to pathology for medical students is also decreasing as it is no longer taught as a stand-alone basic science course during the first 2 years of medical school. Unfortunately, while breaking down barriers between the basic and clinical sciences, this approach has helped to make pathology a poorly understood specialty. Very few medical students have ever seen an autopsy before graduating from medical school [85]. It is no wonder that they are not well equipped to inform and counsel their patients on requesting an autopsy. The declining autopsy rate also creates a negative cycle with unfamiliar clinicians seeking consent in fewer cases. To confound matters, the autopsy, a medical procedure, is costly and not an economic priority in pathology departments.

So where do we see the future of autopsy pathology? The advances in imaging modalities have led to the false perception that the autopsy will be unable to add any additional information regarding a deceased patient's clinical condition [80]. Radiography complements the autopsy but is certainly no replacement for all the autopsy can accomplish. The autopsy remains the gold standard of quality assurance and public health [81]. Though human anatomy remains unchanged over the millennia, insults to the human body do change with time. These insults include toxicities, harmful social trends, changes in cultures with negative body image and expectations, novel instruments of violence, social changes, environmental conditions, and microbiological mutations, and the list goes on. Such changes/insults and their effects on the human body can only thoroughly be appreciated, followed, studied, and eventually prevented through the autopsy. Only by correlating the "world" as we currently understand it with its effects on the human body can we learn and move forward. The autopsy will always be part of the ultimate answer to health-related questions. If conducted thoroughly using appropriate techniques and incorporating knowledge of those often-challenging populations, the autopsy will continue to contribute to science, medicine, and public health.

References

1. Sanchez H. Historical perspective on the autopsy. In: Collins KA, editor. Chapter 2 in autopsy performance and reporting. 3rd ed. Northfield: College of American Pathologists Press; 2017. p. 17–22.
2. Collins KA, Cina SJ, Hooper JE. Getting the most out of the autopsy: ancillary studies. In: Collins KA, editor. Chapter 28 in autopsy performance and reporting. 3rd ed. Northfield/Illinois: College of American Pathologists; 2017.
3. Belsey SL, Flanagan RJ. Postmortem biochemistry update: current applications. J Forensic Legal Med. 2016;40:49–57.
4. Collins KA. Postmortem vitreous analyses. NewsPath. updated 2016. https://emedicine.medscape.com/article/1966150-overview.
5. Palmiere C. Postmortem diagnosis of diabetes mellitus and its complications. Croat Med J. 2015;56:181–93.
6. Elisaf M, Milionis H, Siamopoulos KC. Hypomagnesemic hypokalemia and hypocalcemia: clinical and laboratory characteristics. Miner Electrolyte Metab. 1997;23(2):105–12.
7. Elisaf M, Liberopoulos E, Bairaktari E, Siamopoulos K. Hypokalemia in alcoholic patients. Drug Alcohol Rev. 2002;21(1):73–6.
8. Elisaf M, Merkouropoulos M, Tsianos EV, Siamopoulos KC. Pathogenetic mechanisms of hypomagnesemia in alcoholic patients. J Trace Elem Med Biol. 1995;9(4):210–4.
9. Girard C, Scarpelli MP, Tettamanti C, Palmiere C. Postmortem evaluation of cholesterol, triglyceride, and apolipoprotein levels. Int J Legal Med. 2017;131(6):1777–82.
10. Schirripa ML, Scarpelli MP, Palmiere C. Mediators of inflammation of asthma: a forensic perspective. Am J Forensic Med Pathol. 2017;38(2):153–8.
11. Palmiere C, Bardy D, Mangin P, Werner D. Postmortem diagnosis of unsuspected diabetes mellitus. Forensic Sci Int. 2013;226(1–3):160–7.

12. Khuu HM, Robinson CA, Brissie RM, Konrad RJ. Postmortem diagnosis of unsuspected diabetes mellitus established by determination of decedent's hemoglobin A1c level. J Forensic Sci. 1999;44(3):643–6.
13. Palmiere C, Augsburger M. The postmortem diagnosis of alcoholic ketoacidosis. Alcohol Alcohol. 2014;49(3):271–81.
14. Collins KA. In: Collins KA, editor. Special procedures appendix in special autopsy dissections step-by-step diagrams. Northfield: College of American Pathologists Press; 2010. p. 46–8.
15. Low Blood Pressure (Hypotension). Mayo clinic. www.mayoclinic.org/diseases-conditions. Mayo foundation for medical education and research, 2018. Accessed 21 Mar 2018.
16. Maggio PM. Sepsis and septic shock. Merck manual. www.merckmanuals.com/professional/critical-care-medicine/sepsis-and-septic-shock. Accessed 21 Mar 2018.
17. Singer M, Deutschman CS, Seymour CW, et al. The third international consensus definitions for sepsis and septic shock (sepsis-3). JAMA. 2016;315:801–10.
18. Marik PE, Abdalsamih MT. SIRS, qSOFA, and new sepsis definitions. J Thorac Dis. 2017;9(4):943–5.
19. Kaukonen KM, Bailey M, Pilcher D, Cooper DJ, Bellomo R. Systemic inflammatory response syndrome criteria in defining severe sepsis. N Engl J Med. 2015;372:1629–38.
20. Kaukonen KM, Bailey M, Suzuki S, Pilcher D, Cooper DJ, Bellomo R. Mortality related to severe sepsis and septic shock among critically ill patients in Australia and New Zealand, 2000–2012. JAMA. 2014;311(3):1308–16.
21. Peach BC. Implications of the new sepsis definition on research and practice. J Crit Care. 2017;38:259–62.
22. Balk RA. Systemic inflammatory response syndrome (SIRS): where did it come from and is it still relent today? Virulence. 2014;5(1):20–6.
23. Simpson SQ. New sepsis criteria: a change we should not make. Chest. 2016;149(5):1117–8.
24. Bell M, Collins KA. Postmortem microbiologic testing. In: Collins KA, editor. Chapter 29 in autopsy performance and reporting. 3rd ed. Northfield: College of American Pathologists Press; 2017.
25. Riedel S. The value of the postmortem microbiology cultures. J Clin Microbiol. 2014;52(4):1028–32.
26. Tsokos M, Puschel K. Postmortem bacteriology in forensic pathology: diagnostic value and interpretation. Legal Med. 2001;3:15–22.
27. Carpenter HM, Wilkins RM. Autopsy bacteriology: review of 2,033 cases. Arch Pathol. 1964;77:73–81.
28. Morris JA, Harrison LM, Partridge SM. Practical and theoretical aspect of postmortem bacteriology. Curr Diagn Pathol. 2007;13:65–74.
29. Kavita I, Michael G, Jie W, Jaime G, Jerome L, Joseph L, Tao H. Identification of Bacteria in formalin-fixed, paraffin-embedded heart valve tissue via 16S rRNA gene nucleotide sequencing. J Clin Microbiol. 2006;44(7):2609–11.
30. Martinez RM. Genes in your tissue: probe identification and sequencing microbial targets from formalin-fixed, paraffin-embedded tissue. Clin Microbiol Newslett. 2014;36(18):139–47.
31. Rapid Influenza Diagnostic Tests. Centers for disease control and prevention, national center for immunization and respiratory diseases (NCIRD), Center for Disease Control and Prevention (CDC) Atlanta. https://www.cdc.gov/flu/professionals/diagnosis/clinician_guidance_ridt.htm. Last accessed 2018.
32. DeBiasi RL, Tyler KL. Molecular methods for diagnosis of viral encephalitis. Clin Microbiol Rev. 2004;17(4):903–25.
33. Hans R, Marwaha N. Nucleic acid testing-benefits and constraints. Asian J Transfus Sci. 2014;8(1):2–3.
34. Lucia HL, Kangwanpong D. Identification of dengue virus-infected cells in paraffin-embedded tissue using in situ polymerase chain reaction and DNA hybridization. J Virol Methods. 1994;48(1):1–8.

35. Health, United States 2016. Table 20. US department of health and human services, center for disease control and prevention. National Center for Health Statistics. May 2017. DHHS Publication No. 2017–1232.
36. Collins KA, Presnell SE. Elder neglect and the pathophysiology of aging. Am J Forensic Med Pathol. 2007;28(2):157–62.
37. Collins KA. Elder Abuse. In: Seigel JA, Saukko PJ, editors. Chapter 171 in encyclopedia of forensic sciences. 2nd ed. Waltham: Elsevier Publishing; 2013.
38. Collins KA. The underweight elder: maltreatment, self-neglect, or normal aging? Acad Forensic Pathol. 2013;3(1):40–5.
39. Howe JA, Collins KA, King PS, Yeoman C. Investigation of elder deaths. Acad Forensic Pathol. 2014;4(3):290–304.
40. Collins KA. The negative older adult autopsy: why do they die? Acad Forensic Pathol. 2015;5(1):83–90.
41. Collins KA. Elder maltreatment. In: Payne-James J, Byard RW, editors. Chapter 161 in encyclopedia of forensic and legal medicine. 2nd ed. Waltham: Elsevier; 2014.
42. National Pressure Ulcer Advisory Panel (NPUAP) announces a change in terminology from pressure ulcer to pressure injury and updates the stages of pressure injury. NPUAP, 13 Apr 2016.
43. Tajiri K, Shimizu Y. Liver physiology and liver diseases in the elderly. World J Gastroenterol. 2013;19(46):8459–67.
44. Hoyert DL, Xu J. Deaths: preliminary data for 2011. Natl Vital Stat Rep. 2012;61:1–52.
45. The health effects of overweight and obesity. Center for disease control and prevention. www.cdc.gov/healthyweight/effects/index.html. Accessed 21 Mar 2018.
46. NHLBI. 2013. Managing overweight and obesity in adults: systematic evidence review from the obesity expert panel. www.nhlbi.nih.gov/sites/www.nhlbi.nih.gov/files/obesity-evidence-review.pdf.
47. Clinical guidelines on the identification, evaluation, and treatment of overweight and obesity in adults. www.nhlbi.nih.gov/files/docs/guildelines/ob_gdlns.pdf. Accessed 21 Mar 2018.
48. Bhaskaran K, Douglas I, Forbes H, dos-Santos-Silva I, Leon Dam Smeeth L. Body-mass index and risk of 22 specific cancers: a population-based cohort study of 5.24 million UK adults. Lancet. 2014;384(9945):755–65.
49. Overweight and obesity fact sheet. World Health Organization. February 2018. www.who.int/mediacentre/factsheets/fs311en.
50. Dietz WH, Bellizzi MC. Introduction: the use of BMI to assess obesity in children. Am J Clin Nutr. 1999;70(suppl):123s–5s.
51. Guo SS, Roche AF, Chumlea WC, Gardner JD, Siervogel RM. The predictive value of childhood body mass index values for overweight at age 35 years. Am J Clin Nutr. 1994;59:810–9.
52. Hammer LD, Kraemer HC, Wilson DM, Ritter PL, Dornbusch SM. Standardized percentile curves of body mass index for children and adolescents. Am J Dis Child. 1991;145:259–63.
53. Himes JH, Dietz WH. Guidelines for overweight in adolescent preventive services: recommendations from an expert committee. Am J Clin Nutr. 1994;59:307–16.
54. Keys A, Fidanza F, Karvonen MJ, Kimura N, Taylor HL. Indices of relative weight and obesity. J Chronic Dis. 1972;25:329–43.
55. Petrobelli A, Faith MS, Allison DB, Gallagher D, Chiumello G, Heymsfield SB. Body mass index as a measure of adiposity among children and adolescents: a validation study. J Pediatr. 1998;132:204–10.
56. CDC table for calculated body mass index values for selected heights and weights for ages 2 to 20. http://www.cdc.gov/nccdphp/dnpa/bmi/00binaries/bmi-tables.pdf.
57. Khaodhiar L, McCowen KC, Blackburn GL. Obesity and its comorbid conditions. Clin Cornerstone. 1999;2(3):17–31.
58. Mandel R, Loeffler AG, Salamat S, Fritsch MK. Organ weight changes associated with body mass index determined from a medical autopsy population. Am J Forensic Med Pathol. 2012;33(4):382–9.
59. National health and nutrition examination survey. NCHS fact sheet. December 2017. National Center for Health Statistics 2017.

60. Peeters A, Barendregt JJ, Willekens F, Mackkenbach JP, Mamun AA, Bonneux L. Obesity in adulthood and it consequences for life expectancy: a life-table analysis. Ann Intern Med. 2003;138:24–32.
61. Strawbridge WJ, Wallagen MI, Sherma SJ. New NHLBI clinical guidelines for obesity and overweight: will they promote health? Am J Pub Health. 2000;90:340–3.
62. Golay A, Ybarra J. Link between obesity and type 2 diabetes. Best Pract Res Clin Endocrinol Metab. 2005;19(4):649–63.
63. Jauregui-Garrido B, Jauregui-Lobera I. Sudden death in eating disorders. Vasc Health Risk Manag. 2012;8:91–8.
64. Hewitt PL, Coren S, Steel GD. Death from anorexia nervosa: age span and sex differences. Aging Ment Health. 2001;5(1):41–6.
65. Ratnasuriya RH, Eisler I, Szmuhter GL, Russell GF. Anorexia nervosa: outcome and prognostic factors after 20 years. Br J Psychiatry. 1991;158:495–502.
66. Hudson JI, Hiripi E, Pope HG, Kessler RC. The prevalence and correlates of eating disorders in the national comorbidity survey replications. Biol Psychiatry. 2007;61(3):348–58.
67. Le Grange D, Swanson SA, Crow SJ, Merikangas KR. Eating disorder not otherwise specified presentation in the US population. Int J Eat Disord. 2012;45(5):711–8.
68. Arcelus J, Mitchell AJ, Wales J, Nielsen S. Mortality rates in patients with anorexia nervosa and other eating disorders: a meta-analysis of 36 studies. Arch Gen Psychiatry. 2011;68(7):724–31.
69. Citrome L. Binge eating disorder and comorbid conditions: differential diagnosis and implications for treatment. Clin Psychiatry. 2017;78(suppl 1):9–13.
70. Marques L, Alegria M, Becker AE, Chen C, Fang A, Chosak A, Diniz JB. Comparative prevalence, correlates of impairment, and service utilization for eating disorders across US ethnic groups: implications for reducing ethnic disparities in health care access for eating disorders. Int J Eat Disord. 2011;44(5):412–20.
71. Rushing JM, Jones LE, Carney C. Bulimia nervosa: a primary care review. Prim Care Companion J Clin Psychiatry. 2003;5(5):217–24.
72. Smink FRE, van Hoeken D, Hoek HW. Epidemiology for eating disorders: incidence, prevalence and mortality rates. Curr Psychiatry Rep. 2012;14(4):406–14.
73. Ouellette JD. Statistic on Bulimia. http://www.mirror-mirror.org/bulimia/statistics-on-bulimia.htm. Accessed 21 Mar 2018.
74. Frati P, Busardo FP, Cipolloni L, De Dominicis E, Fineschi V. Anabolic androgenic steroid (AAS) related deaths: autoptic, histopathological and toxicological findings. Curr Neuropharmacol. 2015;13:146–59.
75. Turillazzi E, Perilli G, Di Paolo M, Neri M, Riezzo I, Fineschi V. Side effects of AAS abuse: an overview. Mini Rev Med Chem. 2011;11(5):374–89.
76. Montisci M, El Mazloum R, Cecchetto G, Terranova C, Ferrara SD, Thiene G, Basso C. Anabolic steroids abuse and cardiac death in athletes: morphological and toxicological findings in four fatal cases. Forensic Sci Int. 2012;217(1–3):e13–8.
77. Kutscher EC, Lund BC, Perry PJ. Anabolic steroids: a review for the clinician. Sports Med. 2002;32(5):285–96.
78. Anabolic steroids. National Institute on drug abuse. National Institutes of Health. US Department of Health and Human Services. 2016. www.drugabuse.gov.
79. Solimini R, Rotolo MC, Mastrobattista L, Mortali C, Minutillo A, Pichini S, PAcifici R, Palmi L. Hepatotoxicity associated with illicit use of anabolic androgenic steroids in doping. Eur Rev Med Pharmocol Sci. 2017;21:7–16.
80. Shojania KG, Burton EC, McDonald KM, Goldman L. Changes in rates of autopsy-detected errors over time. JAMA. 2003;289:2849–56.
81. Burton EC. The autopsy: a professional responsibility in assuring quality of care. Am J Med Qual. 2002;17:56–60.
82. Collins KA. Beyond the autopsy: special procedures performed postmortem. Acad Forensic Pathol. 2015;5(2):280–90.
83. Bean SM, Nagler A, Buckley PJ. What are the pathology education requirements for all nonpathology ACGME-accredited programs in an academic center? Am J Clin Pathol. 2012;138:327–31.

84. Oluwasola OA, Fawole OI, Otegbayo AJ, Ogun GO, Adebamowo CA, Bamigboye AE. The autopsy: knowledge, attitude, and perceptions of doctors and relatives of the deceased. Arch Pathol Lab Med. 2009;133:78–82.
85. O'Grady G. Death of the teaching autopsy. BMJ. 2003;327(7418):802–3.
86. Hull MJ, Nazarian RM, Wheeler AE, et al. Resident physician opinions on autopsy importance and procurement. Hum Pathol. 2007;38:342–50.
87. Harrington DE, Sayre EA. Managed care and measuring medical outcomes: did the rise of HOMs contribute to the fall in the autopsy rate? Soc Sci Med. 2010;70:191–8.
88. Lowe JA, Davis CJ. Need we revive falling autopsy rates? PAS Rep. 1977;15:1–7.
89. McPhee SJ, Bottles K. Autopsy moribund art of vital science? Am J Med. 1985;78:107–13.
90. Heller J, Friedlander D, Celler SA. Autopsy findings as a modifier of diagnosis related group classification and hospital reimbursement. Mt Sinai J Med. 1985;52(5):311–4.
91. Turnbull A, Osborn M, Nicholas N. Hospital autopsy: endangered or extinct? J Clin Pathol. 2015;0:104. http://jcp.bmj.com/. Accessed 18 Mar 2018.
92. Bamber AR, Quince TA. The value of postmortem experience in undergraduate medical education: current perspectives. Adv Med Educ Pract. 2015;6:159–70.
93. Hoyert DL. The changing profile of autopsied deaths in the United States, 1972–2007. NCHC data brief no. 67. Hyattsville: National Center for Health Statistics; 2011.
94. Hoyert DL, Kung HC, Xu J. Autopsy patterns in 2003. National center for health statistics. Vital Health Stat. 2007;20(32):1–27.
95. Xu J, Kockanek KD, Murphy SL, Tejada-Vera B. Deaths: final data for 2007, National vital statistics reports;58(19). Hyattsville: national Center for Health Statistics; 2010.

The Autopsy in Medical Education and Training

6

Robert D. Hoffman

Autopsy as Historical Apprenticeship

As in a statement attributed to Pasteur, in the fields of observation, chance favors only the prepared mind. The use of the autopsy observation of human disease for the education of students and practitioners has provided insights that have opened doors for the development of many advances in medicine.

The use of agents that interrupt the renin-angiotensin system, for example, is based upon the elucidation of the biochemical interactions of those factors with one another and with their cognate receptor and effector systems. The nature of the humoral factor renin, in turn, derives from the observation by Goldblatt that surgical stenosis of the renal artery in experimental animals released into the circulation a factor capable of producing hypertension [1, 2]. The experiments of Goldblatt were in turn founded upon nineteenth-century observations made by Bright of patients at autopsy who had myocardial hypertrophy and a shrunken kidney caused by renal artery stenosis, observations made long before measurement of blood pressure was even performed in humans [3]. That about one century elapsed between the initial observation and the key experiment that made possible our present understanding illustrates the point that the observer and the prepared mind do not necessarily need to coexist in space or time. Our observations and materials from the autopsy may contribute to advances to be made far into the future.

The autopsy has been a traditional part of medical education, predating the advent of the pathologic examination of surgical specimens for diagnostic and prognostic interpretation, the ability to noninvasively visualize the internal structures of the body, and the understanding of the microbial, immunologic, biochemical, and genetic bases of disease [4]. With each of the aforementioned advances in

R. D. Hoffman
Department of Pathology, Microbiology and Immunology, Vanderbilt University Medical Center, Nashville, TN, USA
e-mail: robert.hoffman@vanderbilt.edu

J. E. Hooper, A. K. Williamson (eds.), *Autopsy in the 21st Century*,
https://doi.org/10.1007/978-3-319-98373-8_6

understanding and practice, the role of the autopsy has necessarily had to evolve, responding to changes in incentives guiding the time and attention of academic and community pathologists, as well as the depth of examination that was possible because of scientific advances. Whereas in the early twentieth century, autopsies were performed not only by pathologists but also by enlightened and sometimes competitive physicians and surgeons [5], in the modern era, many practicing anatomic pathologists perform few autopsies, if any, as a part of their practice. Autopsy remains as a required part of graduate medical education in anatomic pathology, however, where it provides residents with skills in anatomic dissection, including the ability to recognize and handle fresh, fixed, and processed tissues. The autopsy is often the first opportunity that a pathology resident has to take responsibility for the conduct of a complex medical procedure that may require judicious use of laboratory tests and expert consultations that ultimately affect turnaround time.

In autopsy, a resident must review complex medical records, interact with caregivers to understand their sometimes unwritten concerns, and then concisely synthesize findings in the context of current scientific understanding and medical uncertainty. In many cases, the autopsy is the dominant form of exposure for residents of cardiovascular and central nervous system diseases, which constitute important areas of human morbidity that are not often seen in other pathology rotations. Finally, residency training in autopsy provides a gateway for advanced training for a career in forensic pathology, or for careers where autopsy practice is a key component, such as cardiovascular pathology or neuropathology. Training in autopsy is also useful preparation for careers in academic pathology, because of the need to pass along autopsy training to trainees.

Autopsy Education and Autopsies Performed

As the role of the autopsy has changed, so has the number of autopsies performed, particularly outside of the domain of forensic pathology. The decline in the numbers of autopsies, both in community practice and in academic medical centers, has led to frequent questioning about the relevance and future of the autopsy. Such questioning is not new, but has been ongoing for generations. The reader is invited to review a 1956 editorial, "Potential Values of the Autopsy Today," by University of Pennsylvania cardiologist and former Dean, Dr. Isaac Starr [6]. The theme of the Starr editorial was that the rigorous approach to the autopsy appeared to have declined because academic pathology chairs had allowed their attention, as well as that of their new hires, to be drawn by experimental pathology, which could be performed not only in laboratory animal models of human disease but also by the study of human cells in culture through the newly available immortal cell culture lines. At the same time, the number of autopsies in academic medical centers had actually increased to its peak, reportedly because of the willingness of families to contribute to the tangible progress in medical and surgical therapeutics. The autopsy, once a privilege to the education of pathologist and clinician alike, had now become a drudgery and distraction from more attractive and rewarding undertakings. Huge amounts of data about autopsies had been collected by disinterested rote in innumerable report volumes, file cards, glass slides, and photographs that Starr foretold would never be used. Dr. Starr proposed that the autopsy should be simplified to answer the immediate questions of clinicians, without histology, if possible. Having performed research leading to the development of the ballistocardiograph on patients sent for autopsy, Starr saw the potential instead to expand the practice of such research in the autopsy room. It appears that Starr may have experienced some resistance to his efforts.

Responses from leading pathologists of the day came swiftly to correct some generalizations made by Dr. Starr, but, at the same time, the respondents admitted that some of the points raised in the editorial had merit [7–9]. It was noted that changes in the practices of departmental leadership might contribute to the increased emphasis placed by departments on experimental pathology, as opposed to the simply observational skill of autopsy. It was proposed that the devaluation of simple autopsy observation was passed down from chair to faculty to trainees. As a consequence, the caliber of practitioners of pathology at all levels began to decline. Another point raised was that there seemed to be a large amount of information gathered by autopsy which never in turn was used after having been collected. Autopsy technique was felt by some to have become stagnant and excessively detailed. It was proposed that perhaps streamlining the autopsy to restrict its scope to specifically answer the questions posed by concerned clinicians would help the autopsy to regain some of its relevance to pathology attendings and trainees of the day. Others proposed that the time had come for stakeholder pathology organizations to take a more active role in advising pathology leaders about balancing the roles of service and research, as well as to support the role of education in academic practice, since there was a growing perception that academic pathologists had become too busy to teach. The engagement with clinical colleagues that once occurred over the autopsy had begun to diminish, an interaction that was in fact believed to have even more value for experienced clinicians than it did for students, largely because fewer pathologists fully became proficient at the technical and interpretive skills required to master autopsy practice. In the words of one observer, "The main thing that is wrong with pathology is that pathologists no longer teach it."

Evolving Standards for Documentation of Competency in Autopsy

The point of raising the editorial exchange from 1956 is that many of the observations about academic pathology remain true 60 years later. In the face of progressively declining numbers of hospital autopsies being performed, the Accreditation Council for Graduate Medical Education and the American Board of Pathology instituted number-based criteria for the training of pathology residents [10]. Although initially set as 100 autopsies per resident [11], the autopsy requirement was soon reduced to 75 [12] and then 50 autopsies [13], and sharing of autopsies by two residents was also permitted. Several adjustments have been made since then to limit abuse of the system by residents claiming too many lower teaching value cases, such as macerated fetopsies, as complete cases. The necessity of imposing such restrictions indicates that the emphasis placed on quality teaching of autopsy in various programs is likely not uniform.

The existing number-based criterion for assessing competency in autopsy has been perceived as having failed to achieve its desired goals. Some large and otherwise excellent programs do not have enough available autopsies to support the numerical standards and must rely heavily upon local forensic pathology authorities to provide autopsy experience that is beyond the control of the department. It has been argued that simply reducing the numerical requirement might adequately address the needs of large programs. There are anecdotal complaints to the American Board of Pathology about recently board-certified anatomic pathologists, who presumably had met the number-based criterion during residency training and yet were unable to undertake an autopsy when called upon to do so in the course of their practice (Rebecca Johnson, personal communication). On the other hand, recent trainees have indicated in surveys that they find that the amount of time spent during training on autopsy is excessive and that the utility of autopsy training in their subsequent practice is not great.

In one such recent survey, about 50% of new-in-practice pathologists reported that they did not perform autopsies as a part of their routine practice [14]. The question has been raised whether autopsy should even be included as a part of training in anatomic pathology, perhaps better required only as a component of advanced training in forensic pathology fellowships. On the other hand, the sentiment persists that autopsy training provides some unique experiences in anatomic pathology residency training that should be retained, including the opportunity to review complete hospital records in the context of careful gross, microscopic, and laboratory observations, and to communicate interpreted results to stakeholders, including clinicians and the lay public, in a timely, concise, and accurate way. It is also true, particularly in academic medical centers where pathology residency training and undergraduate medical education occurs, that the need for carefully performed hospital autopsies arises not infrequently to account for unanticipated patient outcomes. To incorporate all of the above considerations, the institution of a competency – rather than number-based criterion for assessment of autopsy proficiency – has been called for.

Stakeholders in Autopsy Education

The public, as the ultimate stakeholder, requires medical investigation of deaths, including autopsy, to inform good government and health policy, to monitor the efficacy and consequences of new diagnostic and therapeutic advances, and to maintain vigilance for emerging disease states arising either from nature or from human activity. Trust in the practice of autopsy in the United States and Canada has resided with the specialty of pathology since the emphasis on scientific patient-centered specialized medical education became the gold standard with the Flexner Report at the beginning of the twentieth century [15]. Many organizations serve the public trust in advising and setting the standards for education and practice of pathology, including the autopsy. There is fortunately considerable overlap, particularly among the pathologist members of these organizations.

American Board of Pathology and Accreditation Council for Graduate Medical Education

The American Board of Pathology (ABP), founded in 1936, establishes the standards for board certification of individual pathologists and also participates in the review of training programs in pathology and its subspecialties in liaison with the Review Committee for Pathology of the Accreditation Council for Graduate Medical Education. The Accreditation Council for Graduate Medical Education (ACGME) has as its role the accreditation of institutions and training programs in all disciplines of medicine, including pathology, and sets standards to which programs and institutions are held for new or continued accreditation, including the permitted length of the training programs, which in most cases benefit from Federal funding. Since 2013, the ACGME has monitored the progress of individual pathology residents and fellows in reaching progressive milestones, coauthored with the ABP, which include autopsy practice (Accreditation Council for Graduate Medical Education and American Board of Pathology, 2013). The ABP and the ACGME interact closely in their duties in other ways. The ABP names members to serve on the Review Committee for Pathology of the ACGME and requires that physicians seeking board certification as pathologists complete training in programs accredited by either the ACGME or the Royal College of Physicians and Surgeons of Canada. Among other standards, the ABP and the ACGME have together set and monitored current numerical standards for education in autopsy during training in anatomic pathology residency programs, as well as fellowship programs in forensic pathology, pediatric pathology, and neuropathology. Any change in the standard for documenting competency in autopsy practice will have to come from the ABP and the ACGME.

Association of Pathology Chairs and Its Program Directors Section

Whereas the ABP and the ACGME are responsible for setting and enforcing training standards for individuals and organizations, respectively, the Association of Pathology Chairs (APC) and its Program Directors Section, usually referred to by the acronym PRODS, have among their roles the execution of the required training and the maintenance of program accreditation, according to the current standards set by ACGME. As recently as the mid-1980s, pathology chairs often also served as the residency program director, with other key faculty directing the respective fellowship programs. As the process of maintaining the accreditation of training programs has become progressively complicated, the naming of a separate residency program director became expedient, and thus PRODS was born to keep close liaison between the chairs and program directors. Pathology residency program directors, among other duties, must ensure that residents in their programs have the required experiences to be documented as competent in autopsy practice. The availability of hospital autopsies, the proximity of a forensic pathology facility, and the incentives and disincentives of faculty to participate in autopsy education are all factors that concern the membership of APC and PRODS.

National Association of Medical Examiners

The National Association of Medical Examiners (NAME) advocates for the practice and training of forensic pathology, a required component of the autopsy experience of every resident in anatomic pathology and every fellow in pediatric pathology, neuropathology, and forensic pathology. The work of NAME to set high standards for investigation of deaths that fall under the jurisdiction of government plays an important role in supporting the civil and criminal justice systems. As professional medical death investigators, members of NAME can play important roles in the autopsy education of residents and fellows, particularly regarding unnatural deaths and the collection and handling of materials to be admitted as evidence in courts of law. Members of NAME figure prominently among the directors of forensic pathology fellowships.

Society for Pediatric Pathology

The Society for Pediatric Pathology (SPP) represents a subspecialty of pathology that has close involvement with autopsy education and practice. The investigation of perinatal and pediatric deaths caused by maternofetal factors, inborn errors of metabolism, congenital malformations, and malignant tumors of childhood are important to the training of every anatomic pathologist. Members of SPP are highly represented among the directors of pediatric pathology fellowships.

College of American Pathologists

The College of American Pathologists (CAP) is a professional organization of pathologists and laboratory professionals with broad representation in both academic and community pathology practice, including autopsy. CAP has a strong interest in the education of residents, fellows, and practicing pathologists, providing print and online educational materials. The college performs advocacy at the State and Federal levels to promote the interests of practicing pathologists. Among its committees, the CAP has Autopsy, Forensic Pathology, Neuropathology, and Graduate Medical Education committees that make recommendations to support autopsy education and practice.

Assessing the Current State of US Autopsy Education

A Working Group was convened in 2016 by the Association of Pathology Chairs and the American Board of Pathology with representation from other stakeholder organizations (Table 6.1) to make a recommendation about how to move forward from the existing number-based criterion.

The Working Group in early discussions had to address significant background limitations before proceeding. Although many works about the value of the autopsy and using autopsy-derived information had been published, the present standard of autopsy training in US pathology residency programs had not been addressed in recent memory. It was deemed imprudent to proceed with making recommendations for the future without fully understanding the present state of autopsy residency education. The best source of information about current autopsy training in residency was determined to be the autopsy service directors of residency training programs, a group which had not been systematically polled in recent years.

The Working Group solicited from current pathology residency program directors through email the name and contact information for the autopsy service director for their residency training programs. Requests to 142 residency training program directors yielded 113 named autopsy service directors. The responses from some of the residency program directors indicated that there was no such autopsy service director for the residency program. The 113 named autopsy service directors were then sent an online poll that addressed available autopsy case volumes and case types, the extent of the practice of sharing of autopsies among residents to extend the available cases, standard methods used on the service for prosecting autopsies, the roles of various personnel on the autopsy service in teaching several key aspects of autopsy performance and reporting, as well as the accountability of the autopsy service director to provide information to the residency program director about the numbers and types of autopsies completed by the residents. Autopsy service directors were asked about the practice of teaching forensic pathology and neuropathology on their services. Finally, autopsy service directors were asked about their opinions about the suitability of the existing number-based criterion of 50 autopsies and whether residents on their service were having difficulty meeting the criterion. The survey respondents were asked to self-identify to assure data integrity, but with

Table 6.1 Stakeholder organizations represented on the Autopsy Working Group

Accreditation Council for Graduate Medical Education
American Board of Pathology
Association of Pathology Chairs
Chairs Section (APC)
Program Director's Section (PRODS)
National Association of Medical Examiners
Society for Pediatric Pathology
College of American Pathologists
Autopsy Committee
Graduate Medical Education Committee

Reprinted with permission from Academic Pathology © 2018

the effect that any results obtained would reflect a best-case scenario. Of the 113 surveys sent to autopsy service directors, 66 at least partial responses were obtained, 42 did not open the survey, 4 opened the survey but did not respond, and 1 email was returned as undeliverable. Of the 66 respondents, 28% stated that they were both the residency program director and the autopsy service director for their program.

APC/ABP Survey Results

The survey results provided findings that highlighted a number of inconsistencies among residency training programs in the way autopsy training is accomplished and documented. The number of autopsies available on the main autopsy service varied over orders of magnitude, with one program having approximately 900 cases available per year for residents on the main service, whereas at the other extreme, 1 program had only 14 cases per year in-house, relying upon the local medical examiner office to supply additional experience for a program of 18 residents. The different types of available autopsies likewise varied considerably, with a number of programs, typically those with the highest total case volumes, showing a very high percentage of the total available cases on the main service as forensic pathology cases. Fetal and pediatric autopsies were heavily represented in the case volumes of several programs with low case volumes.

Because the survey was conducted identifying the programs where residents rotated, the sizes of residency training programs could be incorporated by accessing data on the public resource of the Accreditation Council of Graduate Medical Education. Combining the case volume data with the number of residents in the corresponding residency training program, an estimate of the available autopsy cases per resident could be calculated, with the assumption that all residents were in 4-year anatomic and clinical pathology training programs (Fig. 6.1). Because sharing of autopsies between two residents has been permitted for a number of years by the American Board of Pathology for the purpose of documenting the number-based criterion, the extent of the use of sharing was solicited from autopsy service directors as a percentage of total cases on the main service that were shared by residents. Not surprisingly, sharing was implemented in all autopsies in some programs, whereas in others, autopsies were never shared. The reported rate of sharing was then used to extend the number of available autopsies per resident on the autopsy service. Even with sharing of autopsies between two residents at the reported rates, most responding programs were not able to achieve the number-based criterion of 50 autopsies utilizing cases on the hospital autopsy service. It is presumed that such services must rely heavily upon experience at an outside facility, such as the local medical examiner office for residents to meet the number-based criterion.

The roles and opinions of autopsy service directors were examined next. In about 28% of responses, the autopsy service director also served in the role of residency training program director. Of those autopsy service directors who did not fill both roles, the majority indicated that they did not provide a listing of autopsies completed by each resident to the residency training program director. The autopsy service

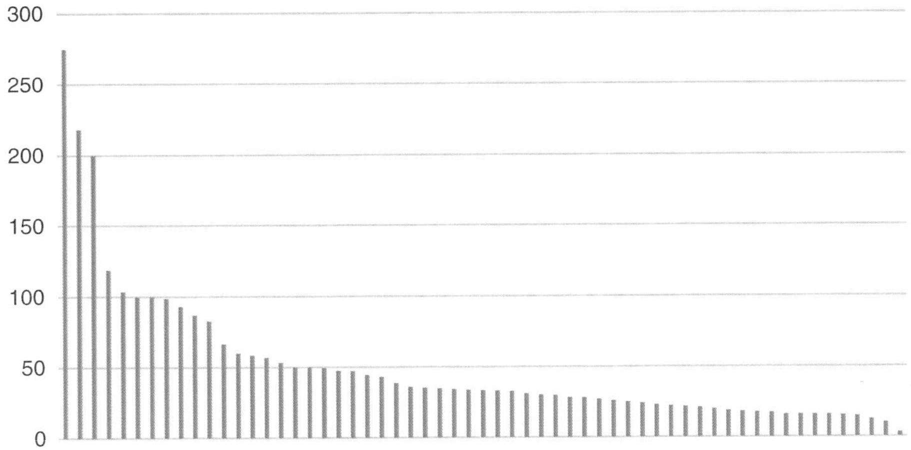

Fig. 6.1 Number of autopsies available per resident by responding program. For each program, the total number of autopsies per year reported by that program was multiplied by four and divided by the total number of residents in the program according to publicly available information from the Accreditation Council for Graduate Medical Education. This calculation estimates the number of autopsies available per resident if sharing of autopsies were not permitted. The order of programs is from the highest available number of autopsies volume to lowest. (Reprinted with permission from Academic Pathology © 2018)

directors responding to the poll indicated a wide range of involvement as the attending of record for autopsies completed by residents on their service, ranging from 100% to 0%. The opinions of autopsy service directors about the current number-based criterion of 50 autopsies per resident were solicited. Although 41% of respondents felt that the present number-based criterion of 50 autopsies was "about right," 7% of respondents felt that 50 autopsies were too many, and 12% felt that 50 autopsies were too few. These data were further resolved by the sizes of the residency training programs, with smaller programs having fewer than 18 residents and larger programs having 18 or more residents. There was a slight trend for directors of autopsy services in larger programs to believe that the number-based criterion of 50 autopsies was excessive, but the results were otherwise relatively evenly divided (Fig. 6.2). Although only 4 of 60 responding autopsy service directors indicated that their residents had difficulty achieving the number-based criterion of 50 autopsies, 3 of the 4 responses came from programs with 18 or more residents.

Entrustable Professional Activities

Because there are many skills related to the autopsy that residents should acquire as a part of their training, and many categories of staff who may participate in that training, the distribution of teaching responsibilities was also examined. A rising trend in medical education is the concept of "Entrustable Professional Activities," defined as those activities in which residents, because of their performance during

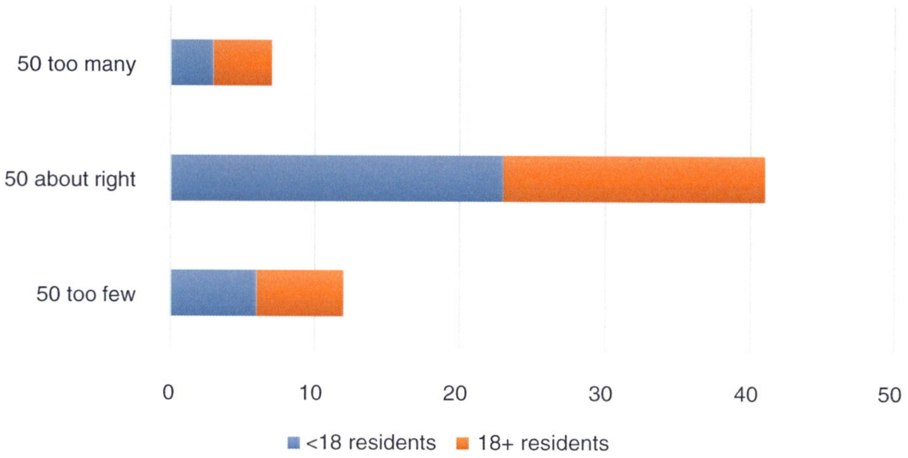

Fig. 6.2 Autopsy director opinions about current requirement of 50 autopsies for resident (58 responses, 8 not answered). (Reprinted with permission from Academic Pathology © 2018)

training, gain the trust of their teachers to perform independently and without direct supervision. Several groups have attempted to identify such Entrustable Professional Activities for pathology in general and for autopsy education in specific [16]. A limited list of possible Entrustable Professional Activities was therefore presented to autopsy service directors, who were asked to describe which type of staff – autopsy service director, other faculty, other residents, fellows, pathology assistants, dieners, or other staff – was most likely to teach each specific Entrustable Professional Activity. An option was provided for autopsy service directors to respond that the Entrustable Professional Activity was not taught to residents on their service. Autopsy service directors were most instrumental in teaching residents about matters of reporting, including composing preliminary and final reports and formulating the cause of death statement. They also were involved in teaching residents to obtain information by interviewing caregivers, to review the medical record, and to evaluate histologic slides. Autopsy service directors played a relatively minor role in teaching residents to open and restore the body and to conduct examination of the central nervous system.

Other program faculty participated most strongly in teaching examination of the central nervous system, review of slides and laboratory data, as well as in reporting. Other trainees, including residents and fellows, were most instrumental in teaching about reviewing patient medical records, performing the gross dissection and sampling, and teaching to review other laboratory information. Other support staff, including pathology assistants and dieners, were most active in teaching about performing opening, evisceration, and closing procedures. Although relatively few instances of procedures not being taught to residents were documented, the most common procedures not taught surprisingly included interviewing caregivers about concerns to be addressed by the autopsy and reviewing the patient's medical record, as well as restoring the body for release and how to extract the brain and spinal cord.

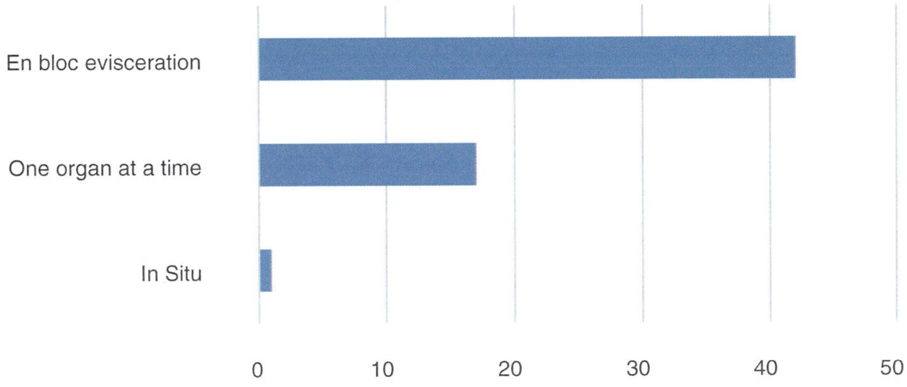

Fig. 6.3 Autopsy dissection technique most commonly employed by programs (60 responses, 6 not answered)

Autopsy Prosection

A significant area of procedural variation in autopsy practice was identified in the method used for autopsy prosection (Fig. 6.3). Although the majority of respondents indicated that the most common autopsy technique was that of en masse evisceration followed by dissection, sometimes described as the Rokitansky or Letulle method, a significant number of programs most commonly taught the method of removing and sampling one organ at a time, sometimes referred to as the Virchow method, with one program indicating that the most common method of prosection involved only in situ sampling of organs. This considerable variation in technical training indicates that programs and autopsy services have varied appreciation of the needs of new medical graduates entering anatomic pathology training to review and build upon gross anatomy skills acquired in medical school.

Recommendations for Autopsy Education

On the basis of the survey, the Autopsy Working Group came to the conclusion that there was so much variation in teaching autopsy pathology to residents that simply reducing the number-based criterion from the current 50 would result in a "race to the bottom" unless an intervention to improve and to recast autopsy education into a competency-based standard was implemented. Toward this end, the Autopsy Working Group discharged its duty by making several recommendations to the Association of Pathology Chairs and the American Board of Pathology.

Autopsy's Importance in Pathology Resident Training

The first recommendation was that training in autopsy pathology should remain as an important part of training in anatomic pathology in US pathology residency programs. Many new-in-practice pathologists indicated in recent surveys that they did not perform autopsies as a part of their practices and that they believed that too much of their time in training was spent on the autopsy. Although based on those surveys there have been proposals to relegate autopsy training exclusively to forensic pathology fellowship programs, the Working Group believed strongly that forensic and hospital autopsy practices are in many ways complementary to one another. Anatomic pathology residents benefit from review and improvement of their gross and microscopic anatomy skills by learning to perform and interpret hospital autopsies, particularly including the exercise of integrating autopsy findings with thorough review of the complete medical record. Autopsy remains the principal opportunity that pathology residents have to see important causes of natural morbidity and mortality in the US population, such as cardiovascular and infectious diseases, which are not commonly seen in other anatomic pathology rotations.

Role of the Autopsy Service Director

The second recommendation made by the Autopsy Working Group was that all accredited residency training programs should have an autopsy service director, charged with the quality and standards of practice of autopsy education, in addition to those of autopsy practice. The Working Group was concerned that there were several programs where no such director existed. Because the subsequent recommendations create important responsibilities regarding the autopsy training of residents, it was determined that those responsibilities necessarily must reside with a member of the faculty who possesses a defined portfolio [17]. At a minimum, the autopsy service director must be certified by the American Board of Pathology in anatomic pathology and have recent experience in autopsy pathology. The autopsy service director must show diplomatic ability to resolve disputes with fairness. An unwavering belief in the value of the autopsy as it improves medical practice and public health is important. From these minimum requirements flow other important roles. The autopsy service director needs to assume responsibility for all aspects of autopsy education as a hands-on teacher, serving as a role model and mentor in autopsy practice and reporting for trainees and faculty. The service director must have a record of competence in technical details of evisceration and dissection, as well as proper documentation and presentation of gross and microscopic autopsy findings. Sensitivity to cultural differences in practices related to death must be observed. A scholarly interest in autopsy as well as experience in participation in multidisciplinary research related to autopsy is important.

Relationship of Autopsy Service Director to Program Director

To the extent that any number-based criterion exists, the Autopsy Working Group as its third recommendation proposed that the autopsy service director be accountable to the program director to report the number and types of autopsies completed by the residents, either shared or not, in addition to ongoing evaluation of the progress of residents in their autopsy competency. The majority of surveyed autopsy service directors indicated that they did not provide any record of autopsies completed by residents to the program director. To the extent that the residency program director is required to attest to the accuracy of the list of autopsies submitted by a resident to the American Board of Pathology as a part of the application for primary certification in anatomic pathology, it seems reasonable that there be a communication between the autopsy service director and the residency program director in the very common situation where both roles are not performed by the same person.

Standardizing the Dissection Method

The fourth recommendation made by the Autopsy Working Group was to standardize the dissection method taught to residents during training. A method using en masse evisceration followed by dissection, sometimes referred to as the method of Letulle or Rokitansky, does far more to reinforce the anatomy skills acquired by the resident during medical school than do other methods, such as organ-by-organ examination or examination in situ. With some planning of the case, the recommended method allows novice prosectors to proceed with less chance of destroying an important anatomic relationship. If the resident is ever in the position of training an assistant to perform autopsies, the method has the same advantage for the practice of the trained assistant.

Progress Benchmarks in Attaining Autopsy Skills

Beyond any number-based criterion for documenting autopsy competency, the Autopsy Working Group proposed as its fifth recommendation that residency training programs also employ Entrustable Professional Activities (see below) as benchmarks for documenting progress in learning autopsy skills. As a resident learns autopsy skills, the attainment of trust to perform agreed upon component autopsy tasks without direct supervision should be documented. These tasks should include all parts of the prosection from evisceration to closing, in addition to microscopic interpretation and integration of all findings into timely and concise preliminary and final reports. The survey sent to autopsy service directors suggests some possible Entrustable Professional Activities; other stakeholders have proposed similar lists. There is a need to have a consensus before further progress is made.

Finally, the Working Group as a sixth recommendation requested that no change be made in the number-based criterion until after the above changes were implemented. A diminished number may eventually be implemented, or progress may be made to a purely competency-based criterion. These recommendations were received by the Association of Pathology Chairs and its Program Director's section, and a position paper endorsing the recommendations has been published [17].

Autopsy as an Entrustable Professional Activity

The foregoing proposals necessitate significant rethinking of the models used to evaluate and document the competency of residents on autopsy rotations. As with other aspects of medical training for complex procedures, one important criterion for the quality of education is the monitoring of attainment of graduated responsibilities by the resident moving through training. After a period of direct supervision, residents may progress to indirect supervision by their attending or senior resident and then even later may assume the role of providing supervision for junior trainees.

The system of progressive responsibility has already been implemented in some departments, which provides an opportunity for senior residents to act as "charge resident," overseeing the early progress of their junior colleagues. A thorough assessment of the progress of residents during training also requires that training be complete and that residents are able to perform technical and cognitive tasks in a reliable fashion. The implementation of checklists has been introduced in several medical specialties to improve the consistency of patient care and to reduce medical error [18]. The implementation of standardized checklists that include a set of tasks that include not only the performance of the autopsy itself but also the pre-analytic and post-analytic phases of the procedure has been implemented in some programs.

In 2013, the Accreditation Council for Graduate Medical Education and the American Board of Pathology implemented the Milestones for Pathology (Accreditation Council for Graduate Medical Education and American Board of Pathology, 2013), a set of benchmark scales, parallel to those in many other disciplines of graduate medical education, that describes the progress of pathology residents in training across a number of important tasks. Two of the benchmark scales within the Milestones for Pathology are specifically dedicated to the autopsy: Patient Care 4 (Reporting), analyzes data and appraises, formulates, and generates effective and timely reports, and Medical Knowledge 3 (Procedure, Autopsy), demonstrates knowledge and practices that enable proficient performance of a complete autopsy (analysis and appraisal of findings, synthesis and assembly, and reporting). These describe in general terms the expected progress of pathology residents on several of the key elements of autopsy procedure and reporting. Although the Milestones for Pathology have achieved their intended goal of providing benchmarks to document the progress of residents in pathology training and have specifically added an element of assessment to resident progress in autopsy practice, they fall short of providing the level of standardization that was recommended by the Autopsy Working Group.

In recent years, the evaluative model of Entrustable Professional Activities has been proposed in other medical specialties [19], and more recently in pathology [16, 20], as a way to assess the progress of residents in obtaining the trust of their supervising attendings to perform critical professional duties without direct supervision. Specifically, for pathology training, the model of Entrustable Professional Activities has the great advantage over the existing Milestones for Pathology in that Entrustable

Professional Activities can be directed to specific tasks in specific rotations, rather than having to be integrated across all of anatomic pathology rotations or all of clinical pathology rotations, as is the case for the current iteration of the Milestones for Pathology. The Milestones for Pathology are in the process of review for updating. The Graduate Medical Education Committee of the College of American Pathologists has proposed a set of Entrustable Professional Activities for Pathology, which includes a set of specific benchmarks for autopsy pathology. The Autopsy Working Group has produced a more detailed set of Entrustable Professional Activities specifically for the autopsy. Stakeholder organizations including the American Board of Pathology, the Accreditation Council for Graduate Medical Education, the Association of Pathology Chairs, and the Program Director's Section of the Association of Pathology Chairs have organized to plan pilot implementation of Entrustable Professional Activities, which in all likelihood will include application to the autopsy.

Autopsy Training Continues to Evolve

Elevating the standards for autopsy training is not a task that is undertaken for its own sake. The autopsy continues to have applications to the "real world," and it plays a strong role in institutions at the forefront of healthcare. Team-based autopsy practice to integrate clinical information bridging between the classical domains of anatomic pathology and clinical pathology has been implemented to provide comprehensive understanding of the anatomic and laboratory data for clinical colleagues [21, 22]. The autopsy continues to find its place in answering diagnostic questions which did not even exist only a few years ago. The timely diagnosis of emerging pathogens may depend upon situational awareness of unusual case presentations and subsequent close collaboration between autopsy services and government disease surveillance services, as in recent deaths attributed to Heartland Virus, for example [23, 24]. Prompt attention to hospital autopsy diagnosis was also instrumental in halting deaths caused by injections of pharmaceutical preparations with microbial contamination [25] and in bringing those responsible to justice.

Advances in targeted therapies for malignancies have raised further novel uses for the autopsy, as powerful biological response modifiers including checkpoint inhibitors have been shown at autopsy to have adverse effects apparently caused by immune dysregulation [26]. Even in cases of successful dramatic responses to targeted therapies for malignancy, after recurrence of tumor and widespread metastasis, autopsy is a unique and powerful tool to collect tissue from many sites of recurrence, each of which may represent a "roll of the dice" by which a malignant tumor has acquired resistance to the targeted therapy [27, 28]. Close scrutiny of such sets of tumor tissue samples obtained from individual patients who have responded to targeted therapy, but who went on to die from recurrent metastatic disease, has the potential to eventually provide predictive information whereby a second- or even third-line targeted therapy may be employed to block the escape of the tumor from the effects of the first targeted therapy [29–31]. Each patient's autopsy sample set may include frozen and fixed normal tissues as well as dozens of individual metastases sampled as frozen tissue for genetic analysis, fixed tissue for histologic studies, and photographic documentation of the anatomic origin of the sample in reference to the dissected organ block. Planning such rapid autopsies requires an ongoing dialog among the autopsy service, clinicians, and investigators to provide a service for a unique subset of patients that can be provided with advance preparation. Minimizing the delay between death and autopsy has been employed for many years [32, 33] and has provided important information for our understanding of shock at the level of cell injury.

The Future of the Autopsy Education

The foregoing discussion has touched on the relationships of autopsy practice with the actions of teaching departments where pathology trainees acquire not only knowledge and skills related to autopsy practice but also attitudes about the autopsy that define the role of the autopsy in education and practice. Autopsy practice has competed through the years with more lucrative and prestigious activities of pathologists including surgical pathology and funded research. Despite distractions from the autopsy, the role of the autopsy in the practice of medicine has remained important because of its several strengths that have remained unchanged against the sweep of history. These constants should be kept in mind as proposals and plans are made for the future of the autopsy.

The first constant feature of the autopsy is that, despite sentiments to the contrary by many of those just beginning to learn autopsy techniques, the competent technical performance of a routine autopsy is attainable by most who seriously attempt to learn it. The author has been privileged to know and work with not only hundreds of residents but also many skilled autopsy technicians with a wide range of education levels who can not only perform superb dissections but also know to stop and get the attention of a more experienced pathologist as soon as an unexpected abnormality is encountered. Particularly memorable in my experience has been the employment of trained funeral director/embalmers [34], having been successfully established at University of Iowa, University of Kansas, and, finally, Case Western Reserve University, where I came to know the system as director of that service from 1992 to 2009. Many college-educated technicians as well as dieners with primary school education have become technically proficient at assisting at autopsy. With regard to autopsy technique, motivation is all, and I have been gratified over the years to learn that, if offered the opportunity, there is a steady supply of staff who wish to learn to assist in the autopsy room. In recent years, the necessities of cost containment have dictated that serving as an autopsy assistant is not a full-time position on my services, but such a position can be leveraged to provide another set of hands in surgical pathology and to assist in autopsy as needed.

The second constant feature of the autopsy is that, relative to other methods used to access the internal structures of the body, the autopsy is inexpensive in its marginal cost, not requiring provisions for anesthesia, life support, or the opportunity cost required to maintain expensive diagnostic equipment. With regard to fixed costs, maintaining an autopsy room requires less equipment than maintaining an operating room and about the same labor costs for cleaning and stocking as does an operating room. Centralizing the performance of autopsies, for example, in the large teaching hospital of a healthcare system, has been used to extend resources, with the addition of modest transportation costs [35].

The third constant feature is that compared with other modalities, the autopsy is able to recover diagnostic and research samples and implanted medical devices with relative ease. The ability to obtain sets of many contemporaneous samples has already been mentioned in the context of being able to fully document the process by which malignant tumors are able to escape suppression by targeted therapies and may perhaps allow for predictive application of sequential targeted therapies. Although there has been progress made in the use of advanced imaging modalities, particularly for the investigation of trauma casualties [36], radiologic methods do not yield histologic diagnoses that would make them supplant the autopsy for many natural deaths. Although the advantages of radiologic methods to document bone lesions and foreign bodies are clear, radiologic methods have also added new perspectives to autopsy evaluation in cases of drowning [37]. The ability to complement traditional autopsy with tomographic studies remains an area for exploration.

The fourth constant feature of the autopsy has been the archival value of reports and in some cases tissue that may be retained for decades. Proposals for the development of a national autopsy database to improve the quality of health statistics emerged almost as soon as digital computers became available for use in healthcare as a tool [38]. Despite valiant efforts [39], concerns about confidentiality have largely eclipsed the originally intended aggregation of reports from multiple sites and public availability of such a database. This setback notwithstanding, the ability to store and retrieve data from huge sets has allowed autopsy data to become incorporated into much broader data resources. At Vanderbilt University Medical Center, a patient record database, known as the Synthetic Derivative, which includes data from entire electronic medical records including autopsy reports, is automatically scrubbed of all personal identifiers and has all dates shifted by a random constant. This resource can be searched for any conceivable phenotype. The Synthetic Derivative is linked to a corresponding de-identified genomic DNA data bank and biorepository known as BioVU. Linked, de-identified records and genomic DNA are collected and sequenced for patients who opt in at the time of blood collection for laboratory tests [40]. The BioVU-Synthetic Derivative has become a valuable and cost-effective tool for phenotype-genotype correlation with the benefit of containing a growing amount of gold standard autopsy data.

A Final Thought

Despite the dire predictions made for the fate of the autopsy generations ago, the hospital autopsy has nonetheless somehow survived. The place on the stage of medical practice for autopsy has necessarily evolved to accommodate changes in healthcare finance, medical education, physical and chemical diagnostic modalities, and the corresponding shifting attitudes of the lay and medical communities, including the attitudes of pathologists themselves. The need for autopsy services extends well beyond the forensic interests of good government. Autopsy will likely never be financially self-sustaining, but there will be an ongoing need for trained practitioners of autopsy, particularly in academic medical centers. The core values of autopsy to provide timely, thorough, systematic, and concise observations and to allow relatively unfettered application of the most advanced diagnostic methods of the day have persisted unchanged. Ongoing scrutiny of autopsy education to refocus on the core values of the autopsy in a changing environment should be encouraged to support the continued value of postmortem examination in the future.

References

1. Goldblatt H, Lunch J, Hanzal RF, Summerville WW. Studies on experimental hypertension: I. The production of persistent elevation of systolic blood pressure by means of renal ischemia. J Exp Med. 1933;59:347–79.
2. Goldblatt H. Experimental hypertension induced by renal ischemia. Bull N Y Acad Med. 1938;14(9):523–53.
3. Keith NM, Keys TE. Contributions of Richard bright and his associates to renal disease. AMA Arch Intern Med. 1954;94(1):5–21.
4. King LS, Meehan MC. A history of the autopsy: a review. Am J Pathol. 1973;73(2):514–44.
5. Wright JR. Sins of our fathers: two of the four doctors and their roles in the development of techniques to permit covert autopsies. Arch Pathol Lab Med. 2009;133:1969–74.
6. Starr I. Guest editorial: potential values of the autopsy today. J Am Med Assoc. 1956;160(13):1144–5.
7. Burn CG, Klemperer P, Karsner HT, Bohrod MG, Barnett RN, Lev M. Correspondence: the autopsy. J Am Med Assoc. 1956;161(2):175–7.
8. Enterline HT, McManus JFA, Coman DR. Correspondence: the autopsy. J Am Med Assoc. 1956;161(8):749–51.
9. Cannon PR. Guest editorial: clinical lessons learned in the morgue. J Am Med Assoc. 1956;161(8):730–2.
10. The Accreditation Council for Graduate Medical Education and The American Board of Pathology: the pathology milestone project. http://www.acgme.org/Portals/0/PDFs/Milestones/PathologyMilestones.pdf?ver=2017-10-09-125332-590 (2015). Accessed 21 Jan 2018.
11. Sebring RH. The pathology residency review process. Am J Clin Pathol. 1983;80(2):197–205.
12. American Medical Association: 1990–1991 directory of graduate medical education programs accredited by the Accreditation Council for Graduate Medical Education. http://www.acgme.org/Portals/0/PDFs/1990-91.pdf. p. 88. Chicago: American Medical Association. Accessed 28 Jan 2018.
13. American Medical Association: 2002–2003 graduate medical education directory including programs accredited by the Accreditation Council for Graduate Medical Education. http://www.acgme.org/Portals/0/PDFs/1990-91.pdf. p. 216, Chicago: American Medical Association. Accessed 28 Jan 2018.
14. Black-Schaffer WS, Gross J, Crawford JM, Robboy SJ, Johnson K, Cohen MB, Johnson RL. Evidence-based alignment of pathology residency with practice: methodology and general consideration of results. Acad Pathol. 2018;5:2374289518790501. https://doi.org/10.1177/2374289518790501.
15. Flexner AH, Pritchett H. Medical education in the United States and Canada: a report to the Carnegie Foundation for the Advancement of Teaching. New York: The Carnegie Foundation for the Advancement of Teaching, Bulletin Number Four; 1910.

16. McCloskey CB, Domen RE, Conran RM, Hoffman RD, Post MD, Brissette MD, Gratzinger DA, Raciti PM, Cohen DA, Roberts CA, Rojiani AM, Kong CS, Peterson JEG, Johnson K, Plath S, Powell SZE. Entrustable professional activities for pathology: recommendations from the college of American pathologists graduate medical education committee. Acad Pathol. 2017;4:1–9.
17. Davis GG, et al. Report and recommendations of the Association of Pathology Chairs' Autopsy Working Group. Acad Pathol. 2018. https://doi.org/10.1177/2374289518793988.
18. Gawande A. The checklist manifesto: getting things right. New York: Metropolitan Books-Henry Holt & Co.; 2009.
19. ten Cate O. Nuts and bolts of Entrustable professional activities. J Grad Med Educ. 2013;5(1):157–8.
20. Powell DE, Wallschlaeger A. Making sense of the milestones: Entrustable professional activities for pathology. Hum Pathol. 2017;62:8–12.
21. Hébert TM, Maleki S, Vasovic LV, Arnold JL, Steinberg JJ, Prystowsky MB. A team-based approach to autopsy education: integrating anatomic and clinical pathology at the rotation level. Arch Pathol Lab Med. 2013;138:322–7.
22. Laposata ML. A new kind of autopsy for 21st century medicine. Arch Pathol Lab Med. 2017;141:887–8.
23. Muehlenbachs A, Fata CR, Lambert AJ, Paddock CD, Velez JO, Blau DM, Staples JE, Karlekar MB, Bhatnagar J, Nasci RS, Zaki SR. Heartland virus-associated death in Tennessee. Clin Infect Dis. 2014;59(6):845–50.
24. Fill MMA, Compton ML, McDonald EC, Moncayo AC, Dunn JR, Schaffner W, Bhatnagar J, Zaki SR, Jones TF, Shieh WJ. Novel clinical and pathologic findings in a heartland virus-associated death. Clin Infect Dis. 2017;64:510–2.
25. Petit AC, Kropski JA, Castilho JL, Schmitz JE, Rauch CA, Mobley BC, Wang XJ, Spires SS, Pugh ME. The index case for the fungal meningitis outbreak in the United States. N Engl J Med. 2012;367:2119–25.
26. Johnson DB, Balko JM, Compton ML, Chalkias S, Gorham J, Xu Y, Hicks M, Puzanov I, Alexander MR, Bloomer TL, Becker JR, Slosky DA, Phillips EJ, Pilkington MA, Craig-Owens L, Kola N, Plautz G, Reshef DS, Deutsch JS, Deering RP, Olenchock BA, Lichtman AH, Roden DM, Seidman CE, Koralnik IJ, Seidman JG, Hoffman RD, Taube JM, Diaz LA, Anders RA, Sosman JA, Moslehi JJ. Fulminant myocarditis with combination immune checkpoint blockade. N Engl J Med. 2016;375:1749–55.
27. Lovly CM, Pao W. Escaping ALK inhibition: mechanisms of and strategies to overcome resistance. Sci Transl Med. 2012;4:120ps2.
28. Dragani TA, Castells A, Kulasignam V, Diamandis EP, Earl H, Iams WT, Lovly CM, Sedelaar JPM, Schalken JA. Major milestones in translational oncology. BMC Med. 2016;14:110–22.
29. Hooper JE, Schneider J. Rapid autopsy and collaboration: opening investigative pathways for research teams. Lab Investig. 2017;97:6A.
30. Alabran JL, Hooper JE, Hill M, Smith SE, Spady KK, Davis LE, Peterson LS, Malempati S, Ryan CW, Acosta R, Spunt SL, Keller C. Overcoming autopsy barriers in the pediatric Cancer research. Pediatr Blood Cancer. 2013;60:204–7.
31. Gorin MA, Rowe SP, Hooper JE, Kates M, Hammers HJ, Szabo Z, Pomper MG, Allaf ME. PSMA-targeted ^{18}F-DCFPyL PET/CT imaging of clear cell renal cell carcinoma: results from a rapid autopsy. Eur Urol. 2017;71:145–9.
32. Trump BF, Valigorsky JM, Dees JH, Merguer WJ, Kim KM, Jones RT, Pendergrass RE, Garbus J, Cowley RA. Cellular change in human disease: a new method of pathological analysis. Hum Pathol. 1973;4(1):89–109.
33. Trump BF, Valigorsky JM, Jones RT, Merguer WJ, Garcia JH, Cowley RA. The application of Electron microscopy and cellular biochemistry to the autopsy: observations on cellular changes in human shock. Hum Pathol. 1975;6(4):499–516.
34. Carter JR, Martin DL. A pathology assistant program: the role of licensed morticians. Am J Clin Pathol. 1970;53:26–31.

35. Trelstad RL, Amenta PS, Foran DJ, Smilow PC. The role for regional autopsy centers in the evaluation of covered deaths: survey of opinions of US and Canadian chairs of pathology and major health insurers in the United States. Arch Pathol Lab Med. 1996;120(8):753–8.
36. Bolliger SA, Thali MJ. Imaging and virtual autopsy: looking back and forward. Phil Trans R Soc B. 2015:370, 20140253. https://doi.org/10.1098/rstb.2014.0253.
37. Levy AD, Harcke HT, Getz JM, Mallak CT, Caruso JL, Pearse L, Frazier AA, Galvin JA. Virtual autopsy: two- and three-dimensional multidetector CT findings in drowning with autopsy comparison. Radiology. 2007;243(3):862–8.
38. Carter JR, Nash NP, Cechner RL, Platt RD. Proposal for a National Autopsy Data Bank: a potential major contribution of pathologists to the health Care of the Nation. Am J Clin Pathol. 1981;76(4 Suppl):597–619.
39. Berman JJ, Hutchins GM. Internet autopsy database. Hum Pathol. 1997;28(4):393–4.
40. Bowton E, Field JR, Wang S, Schildcrout JS, Van Driest SL, Delaney JT, Cowan J, Weeke P, Mosley JD, Wells QS, Karnes JH, Schaffer C, Peterson JF, Denney JC, Pulley JM. Biobanks and Electronic Medical Records: Enabling Cost-Effective Research. Sci Transl Med. 2014;6(234):234cm3.

Forensic Autopsies

7

Victor W. Weedn

History of Forensic Medicine

Death Investigation Has Ancient Roots

Although forensic medicine has ancient roots, its evolution has been so very slow that paradoxically it can be considered a new specialty of medicine.

Suetonius (ca 69–122 CE) and others provided the first record of a forensic autopsy by the physician Antistius on Julius Gaius Caesar after he was assassinated in the forum by Brutus and other Roman Senators on the Ides of March, 44 BCE [1]. Antistius determined that of 23 stab wounds, only the second one in the breast was fatal. It has been proposed that the association with the forum gave rise to our present term *forensics* [2].

Credit for the first systematic treatise on forensic medicine is given to Song Ci (Sung Tz'u) (1186–1249) of the Hunan Province in China, for the *Hsi Yuan Lu* (or *Xiyuan jilu*) or *The Washing Away of Wrongs* (also translated as *Collected Cases of Injustice Rectified*), written in 1247 CE, near the end of the Song dynasty [3–6]. Song Ci compiled, corrected, and expanded earlier writings in the manual, which provided instructions on how to conduct medicolegal investigations, examine corpses, and determine the time and cause of death.

Forensic Pathology Becomes a Profession

The origins of forensic pathology practice in the West arose much later, with the development of medical schools and anatomical dissection beginning in the thirteenth century. Shortly thereafter, autopsies were conducted for forensic purposes.

V. W. Weedn
Department of Forensic Sciences, George Washington University, Washington, DC, USA
e-mail: vweedn@email.gwu.edu

J. E. Hooper, A. K. Williamson (eds.), *Autopsy in the 21st Century*,
https://doi.org/10.1007/978-3-319-98373-8_7

Hugo de Lucca took an oath as a forensic medicine expert in 1249 in Italy. In 1302, the first forensic autopsy documented in detail was made by Bartolomea de Variagiana and three others in Bologna on the body of Azzolino degli Onesti; they reported that the reason for this death was internal bleeding, not poisoning [7]. In 1410, an autopsy was performed on the Antipope Alexander V to investigate the possibility of poisoning by his successor [8]. Ambrose Paré (1510–1590) is considered to be the first forensic pathologist and wrote first on traumatic injuries of organs and then *Reports* in 1575 [9–11]. It was not until after Paré performed a judicial autopsy in 1562 that forensic autopsies became common [12]. In 1598, Fortunato Fedele (Fortunati Fidelis) (1550–1630) is noted to have made a career of performing autopsies and giving testimony about them in court and wrote *De Relationibus Medicorum Libri Quatuor* in 1602 (four volumes) [13]. In 1651, Paolo Zacchias (Zacchia) (1584–1659) published three volumes on forensic medicine between 1621 and 1651 entitled *Quaestiones Medico-Legales* (*Legal Medicine Questions*); he is considered by many to be the father of forensic medicine (Fig. 7.1) [14, 15].

The Holy Roman Empire extended into France, and in about 806 CE, the *Capitularies of Charlemagne* formalized death investigation and required

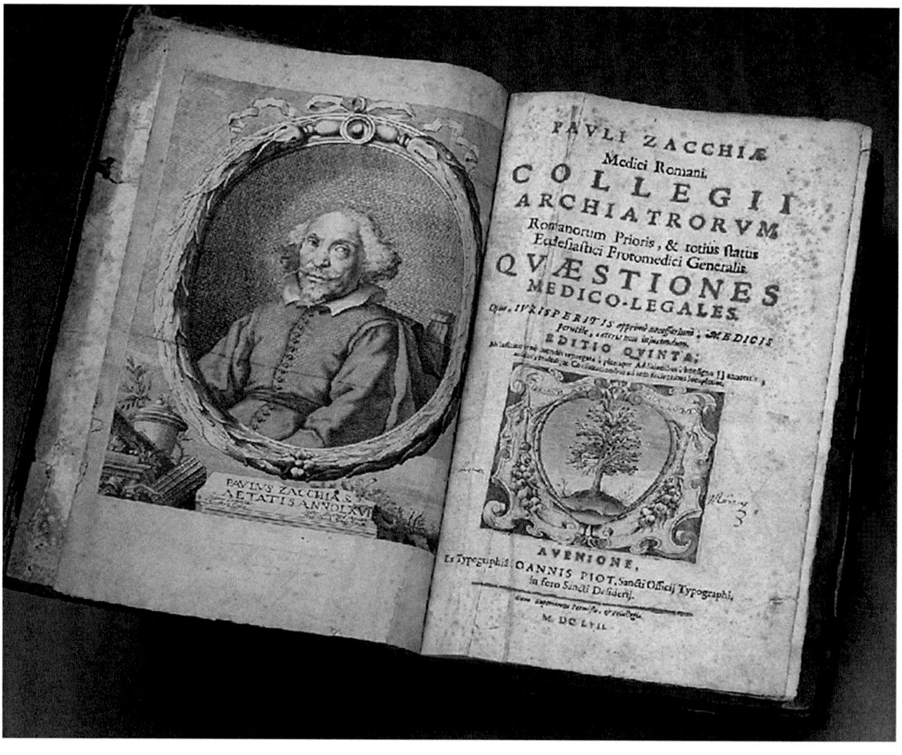

Fig. 7.1 Paolo Zacchias "Father of Forensic Pathology" with page from his published work *Quaestiones Medico-Legales*. https://www.nlm.nih.gov/visibleproofs/galleries/exhibition/rise_image_4.html

consultation of medical practitioners in cases of physical injury, infant deaths, and suspected suicide [16]. The 1507 German *Bamberg Code* required medical courtroom testimony in cases of infanticide, homicide, abortion, or poisoning [17]. Emperor Charles V in the 1532 *Constitutio Criminalis Carolina* penal code (the Caroline Code) extended the practice in all the lands of his empire [18–20]. This led to the development of the medicolegal autopsy primarily by the German Johannes Bohn (1640–1718), who published the textbook, *De Renunciatione Vulnerum Seu Vulnerum Lethalium Examen*, in 1689 [21].

The Enlightenment period of the eighteenth and nineteenth centuries spawned notions of public health, including an interest in understanding why people died, so that informed governmental efforts could help people survive. Throughout Europe, national registries were established, and eventually this came to involve autopsies performed in large numbers to determine the causes of death. Autopsies were performed according to *The Regulations* [22, 23]. Ludwig Casper (1796–1864) and Rudolf Virchow (1821–1902) were prominent in this movement [24–26]. Our current death certificates are part of our national health statistics, particularly our vital statistics system.

Legal medicine (medical jurisprudence) became a separate subject by the seventeenth century, and chairs of legal medicine began to be established in the eighteenth century. Michaelis became the first chair of legal medicine at Leipzig University in Prussia in 1720, followed by chairs in Paris, Strasbourg, and Montpellier, France [27]. In 1807, the University of Edinburgh established the first chair of legal medicine in the English-speaking world, occupied by Andrew Duncan Jr. (1744–1828) [28, 29]. In the United States, although Benjamin Rush (1746–1813) of Philadelphia gave lectures on medical jurisprudence during the American revolutionary period [30], it was not until 1932 that a Chair of Legal Medicine was established at Harvard [31].

England Gives Birth to the Coroner

Investigation of deaths in England developed separately from the European continent, beginning in the medieval period [32–38]. In 925 CE, King Æthelstan (894–939) granted a Charter of Privileges to an English noble, St. John of Beverley, which included a grant of the position of coroner (Latin for appointed by the Crown). This early coroner was a traveling magistrate (circuit judge) who traveled the countryside of the county (*eyre* or *shire*) performing administrative and inquisitorial duties, settling disputes, and levying fines. With time, they became corrupt and lazy, taking years to complete their circuit, and fell into obscurity. Meanwhile, villages were left to the mercy of the greedy county tax collector (*shire-reeve* or *sheriff*), who did not necessarily have the King's interest at heart.

In 1194, Hubert Walter (1160–1205), the crafty administrator of the King, issued the Articles of Eyre to pay for the crusades of King Richard Plantagenet (Richard I, the Lionhearted) (1452–1485). The Articles restructured and formalized the *Justices in Eyre* as three knights and one clerk to be elected in every county as *keepers of the pleas of the crown* (*custos placitorum coronae*). The coroner was elected by all freeholders in the county court and the appointment was for life. The primary charge of coroners was to generate revenue for the King. Newfound treasures, things washing ashore, and stolen goods were documented and confiscated by the coroner for the benefit of the King.

From the very beginning, among other duties, coroners conducted inquests over dead bodies, because they were a source of windfalls for the crown. The estates of those dying of suicide and of those committing homicide would be forfeited to the crown. Objects causing accidental deaths could be taken. These properties could be sold or given to the church (*deodand*). Coroners would also levy fines against citizens and villages that did not properly follow the rules associated with deaths. First finders of dead bodies had a legal duty to raise a "hue and cry," assemble a posse to hunt for suspects, and notify local officials, who in turn notified the coroner. Meanwhile the bodies had to rest undisturbed. If a Norman was found dead, then a fine called a *murdrorum* was levied—from which we get the term "murder."

Another duty of the coroner was to ensure that sheriffs were giving over taxes to the King as they should; coroners had the power to arrest sheriffs. Although coroners often worked with sheriffs, there were tensions between the positions. Eventually, sheriffs, who kept the peace among the living, became the dominant power, and the coroner's role became restricted to ruling over the dead.

Legislative reforms in Britain in the late nineteenth century led to salaries replacing fees as the source of compensation for coroners, positions being appointed rather than elected, and jurisdiction being broadened to all suspicious, unnatural, and unknown causes of death. Further reform in 1926 required 5 years of experience as a medical practitioner, barrister, or solicitor for qualification to become a coroner in the United Kingdom.

American Medicolegal Death Investigation Develops

The American colonies imported the coroner position at a time when the duties only involved death investigation. However, the positions of coroner and sheriff were often combined; sheriff duties were paid by a percentage of tax collections, and coroner duties were paid per death investigated [39]. Colonial charters gave the power to appoint coroners to the governor, but over time coroners came to be elected, beginning as early as 1636 in Plymouth Colony. The coroner inquest consisted of a set number of citizens assembled where a dead body was discovered and sworn under oath to determine how and in what manner a violent or untimely death occurred. The first recorded inquest in America occurred in 1635 in Plymouth Colony. The first recorded coroner's autopsy was in Maryland and involved the clubbing to death of a servant. In 1691, New York Governor Slaughter was autopsied and found to have died of what is now recognized as pulmonary embolism, and not from poisoning, as had been initially presumed.

In 1789, New York passed the first American anatomy law [12]. In 1860, Maryland law authorized the coroner to require the attendance of a physician in cases of violent death. In 1877, Massachusetts replaced coroners with physicians known as *medical examiners*. In 1890, Baltimore appointed two physicians with the title of medical examiner to perform autopsies when requested by the coroner or the state's attorney. In 1915, New York City enacted legislation to replace their coroner's office with a medical examiner office, and this became a reality in 1918, when Dr. Charles Norris (1867–1935) was appointed and given the authority to order an autopsy when in his judgment it was necessary [40, 41]. Arguably, the New York City's Office of the Chief Medical Examiner (OCME) was the first modern medical examiner office. Dr. Norris hired Alexander O. Gettler (1883–1968) as the first OCME forensic toxicologist—also the first within any medical examiner/coroner office [42]. In 1939, Maryland established the first state medical examiner office. In 1944, Dr. Alan R. Moritz (1899–1986), then the Chair of the Department of Legal Medicine at Harvard, coined the term *forensic pathology*. In 1956, the American Board of Medical Specialties recognized the subspecialty of forensic pathology. In 1959, the American Board of Pathology held the first board certification examinations in forensic pathology. In 1966, the National Association of Medical Examiners (NAME) was established [43]. Table 7.1 provides an overview of the ancient and historic milestones in the development of forensic pathology.

Table 7.1 Historic forensic pathology milestones

44 BCE	Autopsy of Julius Caesar
1194	Coroner position created in England
1247	Song Ci, *Hsi Yuan Lu*
1249	Hugo de Lucca sworn in as a forensic medicine expert
1302	Bartolomea de Variagiana, first detailed forensic autopsy
1507	Bamberg Code mandates medical courtroom testimony in certain cases of death
1532	Caroline Code extends Bamberg requirement to the Holy Roman Empire
1562	Ambrose Pare performed a court-ordered autopsy, after which they became common
1602	Fortunato Fedele, *De Relationibus Medicorum*
1621–51	Paolo Zacchias, *Quaestiones Medico-Legales*
1635	First Coroner's Inquest in America, Plymouth Colony
1720	Michaelis named Chair of Legal Medicine, University of Leipzig, Prussia
1807	Andrew Duncan, Jr. named Chair of Legal Medicine, University of Edinburgh, Scotland
1800s	German national death registration, The Regulations (Casper, Virchow)
1877	Massachusetts replaces coroners with medical examiners
1918	New York City Office of the Medical Examiner established (Norris, Gettler)
1932	Alan Moritz named Chair of Legal Medicine, Harvard University
1939	Maryland established first true state medical examiner system
1944	Moritz coins term *forensic pathology*
1956	American Board of Medical Specialties recognizes *forensic pathology*
1959	American Board of Pathology holds first certification exam in *forensic pathology*
1966	The National Association of Medical Examiners was established

The Role of Medicolegal Death Investigation

Today, most death certificates are completed by attending and covering physicians. However, 30–40% of the 2.6 million people who die each year in the United States are referred to medical examiner or coroner (ME/C) offices [44–47]. Of these one million annual referrals, the ME/C jurisdictions accept about half, or around 500,000, for investigation and performance of postmortem examinations or autopsies to determine the cause and manner of death.

Medicolegal death investigation is important to public safety, public health, homeland security, and civil administration. Forensic pathologists will see more homicides than a homicide detective and will be critical to determining the deceased who died at the hands of another—an element of the crime. Forensic pathologists will collect evidence, make significant interpretations, and testify. Recognizing deaths from various hazards resulted in the first driver's licensure law, the first handgun law, regulations requiring certain spacing between slats on baby cribs, and the requirement for collapsible steering wheel columns. Forensic pathologists may recognize a public health epidemic, as they did in the case of the Four Corners hantavirus outbreak, and they also carry out surveillance for bioterrorism and chemical weapons use. Forensic pathologists make identifications in mass disasters. The data they generate assists policymakers; for example, the opioid crisis is defined by the number of overdose deaths, and mortality data will be used to evaluate the governmental response. Death certificates provide insurance companies with the information they need to make payments to survivors.

Many federal agencies rely on the data generated by the MDI system to further their missions and therefore share an interest in ensuring that these data are accurate, reliable, and readily accessible. Death certificates feed into the CDC's National Health Statistics Center's National Vital Statistics System's Death Registry [48]. Local physicians are responsible for completing two thirds of the death certificates, but medical examiners and coroners contribute the other third, which includes the nonnatural deaths (accidents, suicides, homicides, and undetermined). Despite many problems with this data set, it is of huge importance to public health and can be searched by researchers and the public through WISQARS [49]. The CDC's National Violent Death Reporting System (NVDRS) is a more in-depth database run by the National Center for Injury Prevention and Control [50]. The CDC has sponsored such efforts as the Sudden Unexpected Infant Death Investigation Reporting Form (SUIDIRF) to help standardize data reporting [51].

Medicolegal Death Investigation Systems

American Medicolegal Death Investigation Systems

Traditionally, coroner systems are medicolegal death investigation authorities headed by an elected official. However, a few states appoint their coroners rather than elect them. Qualifications for elected officials are minimal; typically, a candidate to run for office must be a US citizen of at least 16 years of age, must be residing in the jurisdiction, and may not be a felon. A few states require coroners to be licensed physicians, but not necessarily forensic pathologists. In Texas, Justices of the Peace act as coroners in addition to their other magisterial duties.

Coroner systems constitute 2000 of the 2400 medicolegal death investigation systems in the United States. Coroner offices are exclusively county jurisdictions and predominate in rural states; thus, they cover only about half of the US population. Coroner offices are independent units within state governments.

The author is critical of coroner offices for the following six reasons: (1) elections politicize coroner offices; (2) elective offices do not allow for national searches and an ability to hire the best person for the job; (3) counties often provide an insufficient population base to adequately fund the office; (4) coroner systems dislink the medicolegal death investigation from the forensic pathologist, who performs the autopsy; (5) coroners are generally non-physicians who certify deaths, not forensic pathologists; and (6) the chief should be a professional rather than an administrator. The National Academy of Sciences has called for the replacement of coroner offices in reports published in 1928, 1932, 2003, and 2009 [52].

Medical examiner systems are medicolegal death investigation authorities in which the chief is an appointed physician—specifically a board-certified forensic pathologist. *Forensic pathology* is the name of the medical discipline recognized by the American Board of Medical Specialties, and *forensic pathologist* is the term for the medical professional practicing forensic pathology. A forensic pathologist fills the government position that has the title *medical examiner*. In practice, medical examiners and forensic pathologists are virtually synonymous terms. However, the term medical examiner is also applied to insurance investigators, state licensure board members, and others. Further complicating the use of the term medical examiner, some medical examiner offices have physician investigators, who are not forensic pathologists and do not perform autopsies; they perform the duties of a medicolegal death investigator as a part-time job.

Medical examiner systems constitute about 400 of the 2400 medicolegal death investigation systems in the United States. Medical examiner offices may be city-, county-, regional-, or state-level jurisdictions. Twenty-two states have a single state medical examiner office, usually in more populated areas of the country. They cover about half of the US population.

Medical examiner offices are sometimes independent, but more often under departments of health and sometimes under law enforcement. NAME espouses the independence of medical examiner operations, even if situated within law enforcement agencies. In *Beecroft v Minnesota* (MN Sup Ct, 2012), the independence of the medical examiner mission was recognized. The New Mexico Office of the Medical Investigator is part of the state university.

Some states have both medical examiner and coroner offices. In many of these states, jurisdictions within the state are serviced either by a coroner office or a medical examiner office. Other states have a state medical examiner office and coroner offices in the counties; in such states, the coroner office provides medicolegal death investigation, and the state medical examiner office performs forensic autopsies for the coroners, who certify the deaths. Examples of medical examiner caseload from three disparate areas of the United States are given in Table 7.2.

Table 7.2 Examples of medical examiner casework distribution

	DC	%	Bexar County	%	King County	%
Population	659,000		1,860,000		2,080,000	
Total deaths	–		13,931		13,898	
Deaths investigated	3063		11,523		12,254	
Cases accepted	1120		2501		2350	
Scenes investigated	712		976		–	
Bodies transported	1222		2408		–	
Cases autopsied	736	66	1470	59	1381	59
Certified as natural	591	53	988	42	940	42
Naturals autopsied	334	55	529	54	501	53
Certified as accident	302	27	897	38	839	38
Accidents autopsied	193	64	486	54	480	57
Certified as suicide	69	6	193	8	293	13
Suicides autopsied	66	96	192	99	254	87
Certified as homicide	107	10	154	7	76	3
Homicides autopsied	107	100	154	100	69	91
Certified as undetermined	34	3	109	5	81	4
Undetermined as autopsied	34	100	108	99	76	94

Source:

District of Columbia Office of the Chief Medical Examiner Annual Reports webpage, accessible at: https://ocme.dc.gov/page/ocme-annual-reports

Bexar County Medical Examiner's Office Medical Examiner Annual Reports webpage, accessible at: https://www.home/bexar.org/medicalexaminer/annual-report.html

King County Medical Examiner's Annual Report webpage, accessible at: http://www.kingcounty.gov/depts/health/examiner/annual-eport.aspx

International Medicolegal Death Investigation Systems

In most countries of continental Europe, medicolegal death investigation is a police function that focuses on suspicious deaths [53]. In these countries, forensic pathologists are generally in academic universities and work as consultants to the police. England and most of the commonwealth countries have coronial systems, although they differ from one another in many respects. These coroner systems are generally independent of law enforcement and make magisterial/administrative pronouncements of the cause of death. In England, unlike in America, coroners must have an advanced degree, and many hold both a medical degree and a law degree. An American-style medical examiner office exists in a few countries, particularly in the Middle East, where there are forensic pathologists and an emphasis on a medical/scientific determination of the cause of death. Medicolegal death investigation offices in some countries may be constrained by the government or religious philosophies. Forensic pathologists in many countries conduct autopsies but leave any histology in these cases to surgical pathologists. Forensic medicine in many countries includes clinical forensic medicine and workers' compensation claims. Forensic medicine in many countries also includes other forensic sciences, particularly forensic molecular biology.

Current Forensic Pathology Practice

Authority for Forensic Autopsies

Hospital autopsies are conducted with the consent of the next of kin and are private affairs, but forensic autopsies conducted in ME/C offices are authorized by statute and are performed in the public interest. Forensic autopsies can be performed over the objections of the next of kin. For example, it would make no sense that a father suspected of child abuse could object to and prevent the autopsy of the child and the potential development of evidence against him. Some jurisdictions permit objection to autopsies based upon religious grounds, but such legislation includes a process to bring the issue to a judge to balance the private interest with the public interest to overcome the objection if need be. Even in forensic autopsies, consent for organ and tissue donation is based upon the consent of the next of kin. A common misconception is that bodies are the property of the next of kin, but in the United States, bodies are not considered property, but rather *quasi–property*, and then family only has a custodial right of sepulcher.

State legislation usually describes the jurisdiction of the office and upon which cases autopsy is permitted and in which cases autopsy is mandated. Autopsies are typically performed in the following situations: the death is known or suspected to have been caused by apparent criminal violence; the death is unexpected and unexplained in an infant or child; the death is associated with police action; the death is apparently nonnatural and in custody of a local, state, or federal institution; the death is due to acute workplace injury; the death is caused by apparent electrocution; the death is caused by apparent intoxication by alcohol, drugs, or poison; the death is caused by an unwitnessed or suspected drowning; the body is unidentified; the body is skeletonized; the body is charred; the deceased is involved in a motor vehicle incident, and an autopsy is necessary to document injuries and/or determine the cause of death; and the forensic pathologist deems a forensic autopsy is necessary to determine the cause or manner of death, to document injuries/disease, and to collect evidence or is otherwise in the public interest.

Medicolegal Death Investigation at Scenes

It is useful for forensic pathologists to physically go to death scenes; however, it is impractical to do so given their heavy caseload, and they therefore depend upon others to do the initial investigation for them. Most medical examiner offices now have their own medicolegal death investigators (MDIs). Some offices rely on police for their investigations, particularly small coroner offices and California Sheriff-Coroner and Texas Justices of the Peace jurisdictions. ME/C offices should defer to the police for criminal investigation involving formal interrogations and sworn statements, but routine medicolegal investigation should be performed by MDIs. As the goals of the ME/C office and police differ, they emphasize different aspects of the investigation. ME/C offices have no interest in the determination of who committed a homicide, while police have little interest in the medical aspects of the case, nor do they have interest in occupational accidents. Medical examiners generally desire independence from law enforcement. Medicolegal death investigators work for the medical examiners and know the information they need to do their job.

In the New York City Office of the Chief Medical Examiner, all MDIs are physician assistants, but the qualifications in most offices are less stringent, and MDIs include a varied mix of retired law enforcement officers, paramedics, forensic nurses, forensic scientists, and morticians, among others.

The American Board of Medicolegal Death Investigators (ABMDI) offers basic registry and advanced certification of MDIs, based upon the National Institutes of Justice Death Investigation Guidelines [54]. The professionalization of medicolegal death investigator community has significantly contributed to the quality of ME/C offices.

Forensic Autopsy Performance

A forensic autopsy is generally conducted similarly to a hospital autopsy and not too differently from autopsies conducted hundreds of years ago. A forensic autopsy involves an "as is" examination of the body as it arrives in the morgue, an external examination after the clothes have been removed, and an internal examination of the head, neck, and torso. Specimens are routinely collected for toxicology examination, for microscopic examination, and for storage for further microscopic examination. A DNA bloodstain card is usually collected and archived. The brain may be retained and fixed for subsequent neuropathology examination and in this case is not returned to the family with the body.

The primary difference between a hospital autopsy report and a forensic autopsy report is the *Evidence of Injury* section. In this section, the forensic pathologist assembles the descriptions of the injuries in a logical fashion. For example, all findings relating to a gunshot wound of the chest are compiled in this section, whereas without such a section, the aspects of the wound might be distributed among separate sections including the skin, chest wall, lungs, and heart.

NAME has promulgated Forensic Autopsy Performance Standards that define what the forensic pathology community collectively believes is a statement of minimal standards for the performance of forensic autopsies by practitioners (Table 7.3) [55]. NAME has also established Inspection and Accreditation Standards for ME/C offices [56]. These standards are in relatively close alignment but also speak to the facilities, staffing, quality assurance system, mass fatality plan, and other office needs. These standards include caseload limits, such that 250 autopsies/year/pathologist is the limit for a Phase I deficiency, but greater than 325 autopsies/year/pathologist is the limit for a Phase II deficiency that will prevent full accreditation. In addition to the Core Accreditation Program, NAME has contracted with the ANSI-ASQ National Accreditation Board (ANAB) for ISO/IEC 17020 international accreditation.

Table 7.3 2016 NAME forensic autopsy performance standards

Section A: Medicolegal Death Investigation
Standard A1 Responsibilities
Standard A2 Initial Inquiry
Section B: Forensic Autopsies
Standard B3 Selecting Deaths Requiring Forensic Autopsies
Standard B4 Forensic Autopsy Performance
Standard B5 Interpretation and Opinions
Section C: Identification
Standard C7 Standard Identification Procedures
Standard C8 Procedures Prior to Disposition of Unidentified Bodies
Section D: External Examinations: General Procedures
Standard D9 Preliminary Procedures
Standard D10 Physical Characteristics
Standard D11 Postmortem Changes
Section E: External Examinations: Specific Procedures
Standard E12 Suspected Sexual Assault
Standard E13 Injuries: General
Standard E14 Photographic Documentation
Standard E15 Firearm Injuries
Standard E16 Sharp Force Injuries
Standard E17 Burn Injuries
Standard E18 Patterned Injuries
Section F: Internal Examination
Standard F19 Thoracic and Abdominal Cavities
Standard F20 Internal Organs and Viscera
Standard F21 Head
Standard F22 Neck
Standard F23 Penetrating Injuries, Including Gunshot and Sharp Force Injuries
Standard F24 Blunt Impact Injuries
Section G: Ancillary Tests and Support Services
Standard G25 Radiography
Standard G26 Specimens for Laboratory Testing
Standard G27 Histological Examination
Standard G28 Forensic Pathologists' Access to Scientific Services and Equipment
Standard G29 Content of Toxicology Lab Report
Standard G30 Evidence Processing
Section H: Documentation and Reports
Standard H31 Postmortem Examination Report
Terms and Definitions

Source: https://thename.org/inspection-accreditation

Death Certification

The primary goal of a medicolegal death investigation is the determination of the cause and manner of death and their inclusion on a death certificate [57, 58]. The cause of death is the underlying injury or illness that results in the death. *Cardiac arrest* is not a cause of death; it is a result of the cause of death. A gunshot wound is the cause of death; exsanguination is a mechanism of death. The manner of death is a nosological classification on the death certificate for public health statistical purposes. This classification includes natural, accident, suicide, homicide, and undetermined. The manner of death is dependent upon the circumstances of death as known at the time of the death certification. Since the manner has a public health function and is not made for a determination of criminal responsibility, prosecutors and courts should not feel compelled to base their case on the certification of the death by the medical examiner or coroner.

Identification of Remains

Death certificates require the name of the deceased and constitute the formal governmental document that a person has died. As such, the identification of remains is a function and responsibility of medical examiner and coroner offices, even though police fingerprint experts or crime laboratory DNA scientists may be used to make the identification. Missing persons investigations are the responsibility of law enforcement. Identification and missing person efforts are interrelated and require cooperation between medicolegal death investigation authorities and law enforcement agencies.

Although many decedents are identified by family or coworkers from the outset, many others are only tentatively identified by personal effects, tattoos, or other means of identification. Generally, formal identification is made within hours or a few days, by family members or fingerprints. NAME accreditation requirements call for x-rays, DNA collection, and odontologic examinations on unidentified remains. Bodies which remain unidentified for 30 days are generally officially counted as unidentified.

The National Crime Information Center (NCIC) is the primary national database for missing persons information that is run by the FBI for law enforcement agencies, but most medical examiner offices do not have access to this database [59]. The National Missing and Unidentified System (NamUS) is a resource accessible to police, medical examiner offices, and the public [60]. NamUS has been key to many identifications. It was created by Dr. Randy Hanzlick, then Chief of the Fulton County Medical Examiner Office, and Steve Clark of ORA, Inc. The National Institute of Justice (NIJ) has contracted NamUS operations to the University of North Texas, which also performs DNA testing of the unidentified remains when needed.

In mass disasters, the primary role of forensic pathologists is to identify the remains. Visual identification is generally considered not sufficient in such situations due to the large number of combinatorial comparisons involved. "Scientific" means of identification, particularly by fingerprints, odontology, or DNA, should be used. The terms "definitive identification" and "positive identification" are frowned upon.

On April 26, 2006, a van carrying nine students and university staff members collided with a tractor-trailer in Indiana [61]. Five people died at the crash scene, including a young blonde woman identified by the coroner as Whitney Cerak. "Whitney" was interred in a marked grave at a funeral with 1400 people in attendance. Meanwhile, a similar-looking woman survived the crash but was unable to communicate, and she was thought to be Laura van Ryn. The van Ryn family kept a bedside vigil over the patient they believed was their daughter. It took 5 weeks before the mistaken identity was caught. This incident prompted Indiana and Michigan to enact legislation requiring *scientific identification* of unknowns.

Forensic Toxicology

Forensic toxicology is critical to the practice of forensic pathology. Particularly in the midst of an opioid epidemic, a large proportion of cases are from drug overdoses. Many medical examiner offices have their own forensic toxicology laboratories, although they may send out cases for further testing, while other offices will send all their casework to a private laboratory.

Forensic toxicology differs from hospital toxicology in many ways. Since forensic toxicology testing must withstand courtroom scrutiny, screening tests are always confirmed by more definitive testing (GC-MS, LC-MS/MS, Q-TOF), the specimens are documented with chain of custody, and the testing is broader, more specific, and more sensitive and includes quantitation. Specimens collected for toxicology typically include central and peripheral blood, urine, vitreous humor, bile, gastric contents, and liver and brain tissue.

Although tables of therapeutic, toxic, and lethal levels exist, these should only be taken as general guidance in interpreting postmortem drug levels. The levels of morphine which can cause death can vary by several orders of magnitude. Whether the decedent is naive or tolerant makes an enormous difference in interpretation. Pharmacogenetics and other factors that bear on the drug pharmacodynamics and health of the individual, such as age and weight, are important to consider. The history and circumstances of death are also important to consider when determining the cause of death. The postmortem interval and the possibility of postmortem metabolism are further considerations. Thus, the forensic pathologist should not overly depend upon drug levels in determining the cause of death.

Mass Fatality Management

Medical examiners and coroners are responsible for mass fatality management in disaster incidents, which include natural disasters such as hurricanes, terrorist events such as 9/11, transportation accidents such as airplane crashes, or others such as building collapses. ME/C offices are also part of surveillance for chemical and biologic attacks and infectious epidemics.

NAME Inspection and Accreditation standards require that the medical examiner office maintains a Mass Disaster Plan (A.7.a), which involves coordination with other local agencies, hospitals, and surrounding jurisdictions. The plan should include sections for chemical, biological, and radiation/nuclear incidents. The standards further require a list of emergency contacts, a list of alternative morgue sites, and that the office engages in disaster exercises.

The ME/C office should have clear guidance as to what triggers mass fatality operations, as well as what would overwhelm its resources and trigger reliance on external resources. NAME advocates that ME/C offices take responsibility for the remains as they are first discovered, which means that the offices should be responsible for the recovery and transport of the remains. If possible, the bodies may be GPS located and diagrammed in position at the scene with the use of a total station. Refrigerated trucks may be used to store the bodies. Operations will normally be split between antemortem and postmortem data collection that will eventuate in the reconciliation and identification of remains. The antemortem data collection will primarily consist of asking families for descriptions of their loved one and what he or she was wearing that day, photographs, contact information for the victim's dentist, and DNA collection. This would typically be accomplished at the Victim Identification Center (VIC), a component of the Family Assistance Center (FAC). Families at the FAC should be daily updated on the operations. First notification of an identification should be to the family. The postmortem data collection will be accomplished in the morgue. Typically, separate stations will be used for triage, personal effects, radiology, pathology/DNA collection, anthropology, fingerprinting, and odontology stations; the remains will be escorted through the various stations.

The National Disaster Medical System (NDMS) is a federal response group run by the Department of Health and Human Services (DHHS) Assistant Secretary for Preparedness and Response (ASPR) for public health emergencies [62]. NDMS includes Disaster Mortuary Operational Response Teams (DMORTs) [63]. Regional DMORTs are composed of forensic pathologists, forensic odontologists, forensic anthropologists, morticians, and others who work in their normal capacities until federally activated to support DVI operations of jurisdictions in need. The DVI team will use their Victim Identification Profile software system to help match antemortem and postmortem identification profiles. Many smaller jurisdictions with few resources and expertise rely on such resources.

NAME published Standard Operating Procedures for Mass Fatality Management in 2010 [64]. Guidelines for mass fatality operations are being produced by the National Institute of Standards and Technology (NIST) Organization of Scientific Area Committees (OSAC) Disaster Victim Identification (DVI) subcommittee [65] and the American Academy of Forensic Sciences (AAFS) Academy Standards Board (ASB) Disaster Victim Identification (DVI) Consensus Body [66].

Medicolegal Testimony

An integral part of forensic medical practice is testimony [67]. The vast majority of homicide cases never go to trial, but are instead resolved by plea bargain. However, when a homicide is litigated, forensic pathologists will usually be called by prosecutors not only to establish that the death resulted from the action of another person as an element of the crime but also to convey to jurors the inhumanity of the death. Although sometimes called upon as an unpaid *fact witness*, the forensic pathologist is usually called as an *expert witness* to give an opinion, which is beyond the ken of a lay person due to education, training, or experience.

Discovery is the pretrial process in which the attorneys produce evidence and make reciprocal disclosures. Discovery includes disclosure of the witnesses to be called and the basis for their opinions. Interrogatories are formal questions which are asked by the court when asked to do so by the attorneys. Orders to produce documents may be issued. Depositions may be taken before trial, but these are, despite their apparent informal nature, considered formal testimony under oath—the attorneys will be looking for inconsistencies between the deposition and the eventual trial testimony. *Brady material* is any potentially exculpatory evidence known to the prosecution in a criminal case and must be disclosed to the defense. *Giglio material* is any damaging information about the witness known to the prosecution and must also be disclosed to the defense.

Before trial, the witness should have a pretrial conference with the attorney calling him or her to give testimony. During this meeting, the attorney should go over the questions and issues of the case. The attorney should not tell a witness what to say but may suggest wording. The photographs and any other demonstrative evidence should be agreed upon at this time.

A subpoena will be issued to call the witness to appear in court. Initially, the witness will be sworn in by giving an oath before the court. Then the witness will be asked to state their name, to spell it, and to state his or her employment position. Testimony will begin with a description of the educational experience of the witness to establish a foundation for the court to admit the expert testimony. The testimony will begin with direct examination by the attorney, who called the witness. This direct examination will call for longer, descriptive answers, in which the expert will give his or her opinion—often with the help of photographs and other demonstrative evidence. The witness will usually be asked to authenticate the autopsy report and photographs that will be given to the jury. The opposing counsel will then cross-examine the witness, often asking yes or no questions. Leading questions may not be asked on direct examination but may be asked on cross-examination. This may be followed by redirect and recross.

Important Cases

The US Supreme Court in *Daubert v. Merrell Dow Pharmaceuticals, Inc.* (509 U.S. 579, 1994), ruled that the Federal Rules of Evidence (FRE) superseded the earlier *Frye v. U.S.* (293 F. 1013, DC Cir 1923) case that held that novel scientific evidence must gain general acceptance in the specific field or community for it be admitted into court for presentation to the jury. Daubert established the judge as the gatekeeper and that she should find the evidence to be relevant and reliable for admissibility. The court articulated a set of non-exhaustive Daubert factors used to judge the reliability of the evidence including the testability of the asserted science, peer-reviewed publication, known error rates, and general acceptance of the relevant community. In *Kumho Tire Co v. Carmichael* (526 U.S. 137, 1999), the Court also made clear that technical expertise could also be based upon experience, even if not scientific.

The Federal Rules of Evidence provide the legal framework by which expert testimony may be given. The Federal Rules of Civil Procedure provide additional guidance for civil proceedings. These federal rules are generally mirrored in state evidentiary codes. In general, forensic testimony must be found to be relevant and reliable, and the bases for the testimony must be disclosed.

The US Supreme Court in *Crawford v. Washington* (541 U.S. 36, 2004) overruled previous case law and declared that the Confrontation Clause of the Sixth Amendment of the federal Constitution makes adverse material witnesses available at trial for cross-examination by the defense. This may become problematic when the witness is not available for trial. Crawford was specifically applied to forensic scientists first in *Melendez-Diaz v. Massachusetts* (557 U.S. 305, 2009) and then in *Bullcoming v. New Mexico* (564 U.S. 647, 2011) and *Williams v. Illinois* (567 U.S. 132 S.Ct. 2221, 2012). The result is that forensic scientists who produce evidence used by the prosecution must be made available when called. However, most state courts, such as in *People v. Dungo* (55 Cal.4th 608 & 982, 2012), have found that autopsy reports are not testimonial in nature, and therefore the original forensic pathologist is not required to testify.

The Future of Forensic Autopsy Practice

Current Medicolegal Death Investigation Environment

Medical examiner and coroner offices are historically underfunded. Policymakers often see funding ME/C offices as a waste of money on the dead, even though they function for the living. As a generality, a medical examiner's office can be adequately funded for only \$3 to \$3.50 per citizen per year [68]. There is not a vocal constituency to strongly advocate for ME/C offices. Nonetheless, facilities and resources are stronger now than ever before, albeit with some significant gaps. So too, the sophistication of the practice of forensic pathology and the quality of medicolegal death investigation overall has vastly improved. Furthermore, expectations have increased as the bar has been raised but also as television has increased awareness and popularized forensic pathology.

The number of board-certified forensic pathologists working in the field is estimated between 500 and 700. This has been thought to represent only half of the number of forensic pathologists needed for adequate medicolegal death investigation across the United States [69]. However, the recent opioid crisis has dramatically increased the need for more forensic pathologists. Between 30 and 40 newly minted forensic pathology fellows become board certified and enter the workforce per year. This is far below what is needed. Of the 70 or so forensic pathology fellowship programs, funding is available for only about half of the slots. Forensic pathology is the only medical training that is not subsidized through federal medical spending, because medical examiner offices fall outside of hospital and clinical care. As of 2017, the

National Institute of Justice has funded seven fellows in the field. Despite CSI, the Kay Scarpetta novels, and other media, there is no clamor for pathology residents to go into the discipline. The forensic pathology community consistently points to a few predominant factors to explain this. The first is the relatively low pay for forensic pathologists. After spending a fellowship year in forensic pathology, a fellow will find that she will make perhaps only half of what a pathologist going straight into hospital practice would earn. However, recently the critical shortage has led to offices hiring forensic pathologists away from other offices and driving salaries higher. The second factor is a lack of exposure of students to forensic pathology. Most pathologists obtain exposure to forensic pathology due to the requirement for performing autopsies during residency, but this requirement has been reduced and continues to be threatened by pathology residency program directors, who perceive it to be a waste. Moreover, there are fewer medical students exposed to pathology, and this appears to be lowering the number going into pathology, threatening the pipeline. Thirdly, in some pathology programs, residents are actively discouraged from going into forensic pathology as many pathology faculty members do not relate well to the field and speak ill of it; most academic pathology programs lack forensic pathologist faculty members.

The Impetus for Change

The opioid crisis that is ongoing at the time of this writing is shining a light on the critical shortage of forensic pathologists in the United States and their importance to society. The opioid crisis is defined in terms of the number of deaths, and the success in combatting it will be measured with mortality data. Every overdose case should be autopsied by a forensic pathologist. Yet surprisingly, the medical examiner community has been left out of the funding to support state and local efforts to combat the crisis—federal, state, and local governmental efforts have focused on prevention, interdiction, and treatment, and medicolegal death investigation is neglected. However, there appears to be the beginning of widespread recognition of the value of medicolegal death investigation in this context, particularly by the Department of Justice, the Centers for Disease Control and Prevention, and among some key legislators, which may lead to support and key changes.

The forensic sciences have recently garnered significant criticism, which may well lead to efforts that may benefit forensic pathology with the rest of the forensic science community. It is significant that the 2013–2017 National Commission on Forensic Science (NCFS) had a Medicolegal Death Investigation (MDI) Subcommittee [70, 71]. So too, the National Institute of Standards and Technology (NIST) Organization of Scientific Area Committees for Forensic Science (OSAC) has a Crime Scene/Death Investigation Scientific Area Committee, a Medicolegal Death Investigation (MDI) Subcommittee, and a NAME representative on the Forensic Science Standards Board [72]. The forerunner to the OSAC MDI Subcommittee was the Scientific Working Group on Medicolegal Death Investigation (SWGMDI), which created numerous important documents that can still be found posted on the web [73].

Beyond these movements, it does appear that the medical examiner community has been slowly gaining ground in terms of resources, respect, and capability, which auspiciously bodes well for still further improvements, even if no support materializes from the opioid crisis or for the forensic science community. As relatively new organs of government, medical examiner offices are still finding their place, and the community has been actively advocating for support for a substantial time. It is significant that the Office of Science and Technology Policy has a Medicolegal Death Investigation Committee that released two reports in 2017 [74].

Legislative Efforts and Proposed New Structures

The Consortium of Forensic Science Organizations (CFSO) is the primary advocacy group for the forensic science community, including the medicolegal death investigation community [75]. The CFSO membership is comprised of NAME, the American Academy of Forensic Sciences, the American Society for Crime Laboratory Directors, the International Association for Identification, the International Association of Forensic Nurses, the Society of Forensic Toxicologists, and the American Board of Forensic Toxicology as members. In aggregate, the CFSO represents 21,000 forensic scientists. Advocacy of the CFSO includes:

- *Mandatory Accreditation of ME/C Offices*: The CFSO, NAME, NCFS, and OSTP have all advocated for mandatory accreditation, which would force at least minimal funding and staffing of such offices.
- *Mandatory Certification of Medicolegal Death Investigators*: Similarly, the CFSO, NAME, NCFS, and OSTP have advocated for certification of medicolegal death investigators, including coroners who function as medicolegal death investigators.
- *CDC Office of Forensic Medicine (OFM)*: There is no voice for forensic pathologists within the US federal government. The Armed Forces Medical Examiner System (AFMES) is the only medical examiner office within the US federal government, and it has not been the voice needed for the state and local offices. A few forensic pathologists are positioned elsewhere in the federal government, but none in positions of substantial influence. The NCFS recommended the establishment of a National Office of Medicolegal Death Investigation, with the unfortunate acronym of "NOMDI" [76]. The CFSO has advocated for the creation of an OFM, headed by a forensic pathologist, within the CDC from consolidating certain existing programs (NVDRS, SIDS), which would be analogous to the current CDC Office for State, Tribal, Local, and Territorial Support (OSTLTS).
- *Workforce Development*: Increasing forensic pathologist manpower has been a top priority for the forensic pathology community, but it is difficult to do. The National Institute of Justice (NIJ) awarded funding for eight forensic pathology fellows in 2017; this program should be continued and expanded. A student loan

forgiveness program would be useful, or at least forensic pathology could be designated a critical area need under existing programs. Granting J1 and H1 Visa waivers for foreign pathology students and foreign medical graduates would help.

- *Operational Funding*: The CFSO has long supported the NIJ Coverdell grant program, which has provided the only federal operational support for crime labs and ME/C offices; however, ME/C offices generally receive only a few thousand dollars, if anything at all. In 2017 NIJ established a grant program specifically for the medicolegal death investigation community for the accreditation of offices and forensic pathology fellowships, which should be continued and expanded.
- *Opioid Crisis Funding*: The CFSO has advocated that some of the Department of Health and Human Services (DHHS) Substance Abuse and Mental Health Assistance (SAMSHA) funding given to states for the medical response should flow to ME/C offices. Congress authorized a half billion-dollar expenditure for the opioid crisis in the 21st Century Cures Act, which was enacted in late 2016, but none has yet been made available to ME/C offices.
- *Research Funding*: The NIH does not fund applied research in forensic pathology; instead funding has come from the NIJ [77]. The CFSO has advocated for the creation of an Office of Forensic Sciences within DOJ, created from the current NIJ Office of Investigative and Forensic Sciences. The OFS would be positioned higher in the structure of DOJ and would be headed by a forensic scientist. It is believed that more research might flow from such reorganization.
- *Model Medical Examiner Legislation*: In 1954, then the National Commission for Uniform State Laws (now the Uniform Law Commission) created a Model Post-Mortem Examinations Act which provided guidance for states to establish medical examiner systems [78]. This model legislation is woefully inadequate, but guidance is still needed for states, which generally have old and spotty statutes. New updated model state legislation would be useful [79]. The NCFS recommended the creation of new model medical examiner legislation [80].

Flowering of the Forensic Autopsy Practice

Autopsy practice has remained largely unchanged for centuries. A number of technologies to augment and advance the autopsy practice within ME/C offices are being implemented or are on the horizon.

Advanced Imaging X-rays are routinely used for unidentified remains, charred remains, gunshot victims, explosion victims, decomposed remains, and in infants to locate bullets, knife tips, and other foreign objects, as well as to document identifying features. The LODOX-Statscan is replacing traditional x-ray units across the United States due to its ease of use, speed, and lower radiation exposure [81]. A few US medical examiner offices have a computed tomography (CT) scanner, and even fewer offices also have magnetic resonance imaging (MRI) capabilities. However, advanced imaging technologies are routinely used in many medical examiner offices throughout the world; this is an area where the United States lags behind. Advanced imaging can be a very useful adjunct to traditional autopsy practice and is sometimes used in place of autopsy, thus increasing efficiency in those offices that use it in this way [82]. Advanced imaging can be advantageous in revealing pneumothoraces and bony fractures; with angiography it will show thromboemboli, basilar artery and aneurysm ruptures, as well as coronary atherosclerotic narrowing and occlusions. Advanced imaging has the potential to directly visualize myocardial infarctions and strokes, if the body is fresh and not decomposed. Reconstruction using advanced imaging techniques permits visuals that are unparalleled for demonstrations in court [83].

Molecular Autopsies A few medical examiner offices have internal forensic DNA identification testing capability, and even fewer have genetic testing capability, but there is a broad need for both. The ability to diagnose genetic conditions may be of great clinical value to families which harbor an unsuspected genetic trait, as with testing for common conditions such as hemochromatosis, sickle cell anemia, cystic fibrosis, Marfan's syndrome, or even multigenic diseases such as diabetes and hypercholesterolemia. Medical examiners should be interested in possible lethal genetic conditions such as cardiac channelopathies, coagulopathies, vascular wall degenerative diseases, and arrhythmogenic right ventricular dysplasia. Pharmacogenomic testing, such as for fast or slow cytochrome P450 acetylation, may help in toxicology interpretation. Whole-exome testing may be becoming feasible, as well.

Proteomic Biomarker Analyses Cardiac markers have not proven sufficiently useful for routine postmortem application to date. Using new high-sensitivity troponins for the diagnosis of myocardial infarction or brain natriuretic peptide (BNP) for the diagnosis of congestive heart failure has simply not been explored in medical examiner offices. Furthermore, mass spectrometry instrumentation has also greatly advanced, and particularly the Orbitrap MS technology may be of interest. It would be important to a forensic pathologist if proteomic profiling revealed a hypercoagulative state, prolonged hypoxemia, or even significant pain (nociception), for instance. The potential for proteomic analysis of the blood to reveal a cause of death is great.

Microbial Analysis Postmortem cultures are notoriously unreliable, due to conditions no longer conducive to pathogen growth and overgrowth from the skin and gut flora, yet testing for infectious agents continues would be valuable. The development of MALDI-TOF and NGS methods of microbiome testing may prove viable here. Microbiome testing does not require continued growth. It is also sensitive to broad commensal patterns that might show either a normal or abnormal flora. Postmortem microbiome testing is currently under investigation to determine postmortem interval, but not yet for pathogen detection.

Fluorescence of the Role of the Forensic Autopsy

The author believes that forensic autopsies will take on an increasingly important role in the future. The hope is that there will be an Office of Forensic Medicine within CDC and an Office of Forensic Science within DOJ which may facilitate the growth of medical examiner offices, perhaps in the following ways:

Public Health Medicolegal death investigation has often emphasized suspicious deaths and criminal prosecution, but the public health aspects have been increasingly important. Virchow performed autopsies on the theory that causes of death need to be known to inform public health policy. It is the medical examiner that has a legal responsibility to investigate deaths and is authorized to examine the bodies. Forensic pathologists as medical examiners can answer many questions that are important to public health, but to date, they have been so overwhelmed with other work that their full potential has not been realized. For example, if there is a concern about an environmental toxin in a community, wouldn't it make sense to test the bodies from that jurisdiction for the toxin? Why is it that most trauma statistics refer to the percentage of deaths of any given trauma once they reach the emergency room, rather than also include the deaths of those that never reached the emergency room? Medical examiner offices should be nodes of a national information network for consumer product safety, for medical device efficacy, and for the safety of newly emerging drugs. Death certificates do function in this way, but there is a great deal of more information that could be obtained and shared.

Clinical Forensic Medicine In many countries outside the Unites States, forensic medical doctors examine the injuries of live patients. In the United Kingdom, they have been called *police surgeons*. In some countries, these clinical forensic medical examiners are the primary experts in workers' compensation hearings. It would seem to make sense that forensic medical doctors, perhaps forensic pathologists, with forensic nurses, would work in centers that cater to victims of child abuse, domestic violence, rape, and elder abuse. Forensic pathology of the deceased should help inform the examination of the living, and vice versa.

Hospital Autopsies Medical examiner offices may become centers for autopsies of hospital deaths. The hospital autopsy practice continues to decline, but families still have a need for autopsies to answer their questions. Autopsy pathology expertise is increasingly in the hands of forensic pathologists. Many forensic pathologists perform private autopsies in addition to or instead of public forensic medical examiner work. Furthermore, if the use of autopsies for quality assurance of healthcare makes a resurgence, as it should, then there is an argument that it should fall to the governmental medical examiners. Currently, forensic pathologists are too busy with their forensic autopsies to worry with hospital autopsies, but this could change.

Biomedical Research As autopsies become more powerful diagnostic tools, they also become more valuable for research. The use of animals for biomedical research purposes continues to decline. With the decrease in wide tumor excision and the rise of liquid biopsies and greater use of cytology, tissue specimens will probably become more valuable, perhaps resulting in a greater need for autopsy tissues (see Chaps. 8 and 9). For all of these reasons, autopsy pathology may take on a bigger role in biomedical research.

For your reference, Table 7.4 provides a list of the most important forensic pathology terms discussed and used in this chapter and their definitions.

Table 7.4 Important forensic pathology terms and definitions

Forensic autopsy – An autopsy performed under the auspices of the governmental medicolegal death investigation authority, either a medical examiner's or coroner's office; it does not require consent of the next-of-kin.
Forensic pathology – The subdiscipline of anatomic pathology, recognized by the American Board of Medical Specialties, involved with medicolegal death investigation—the principle tool of which is the forensic autopsy.
Forensic medicine – The area of medicine devoted to the application of medicine to questions of law and subsumes both forensic pathology and clinical forensic medicine.
Forensic pathologist – The medical practitioner of forensic medicine.
Medical examiner – A forensic pathologist, who works for the medicolegal death investigation authority in the employment position title of "medical examiner." In common parlance, "medical examiner" and "forensic pathologist" are often used interchangeably. [New Mexico uses the term "medical investigator."]
Coroner – Usually an elected official, but sometimes an appointed official, and sometimes required to be a physician, who heads an office which is not required to be headed by a forensic pathologist; most coroners are non-physicians and essentially function as medicolegal death investigators. By contrast, a medical examiner's office is headed by a forensic pathologist.
Medicolegal death investigation – The application of medical knowledge to the investigation of death for governmental or legal concerns.
Medicolegal death investigator – A specialized staff member who works for a coroner or medical examiner and is responsible for investigating deaths, going to death scenes, and providing a short history to the forensic pathologist before performing a forensic autopsy.
Legal medicine – A term once used for forensic medicine, but now more generally used as an area of law pertaining to medical concerns.

References

1. Suetonius (Gaius Suetonius Tranquillus). The twelve caesars (R Graves trans.). London: Penguin Classics; 1957.
2. Hooi LW. Autopsy report on Julius Caesar's death gave rise to the term "forensic" in Latin which means "before the forum", *Bambooinnovator*, 3/13/2014.
3. Smith S. The history and development of forensic medicine. Br Med J. 1951;1(4707):599–607.
4. Tzu S. The washing away of wrongs: forensic medicine in thirteenth-century China, 1247 (BE McKnight trans.), 1247. Ann Arbor: Center for Chinese Studies, The University of Michigan; 1981.
5. Asen D. Song Ci (1186–1249). "Father of World Legal Medicine," history, science, and forensic culture in contemporary China. East Asian Sci Technol Soc. 2017;11(2):185–207. Available at: http://easts.dukejournals.org/content/early/2017/02/08/18752160-3812294.abstract.
6. Fu LKT. Sung Tz'u (1186-1249) and medical jurisprudence in ancient China. J MedBiog. 2004;12(2):95–104.
7. Park K. The criminal and the saintly body: autopsy and dissection in Renaissance Italy. Renaissance Quarterly. 1994;47(1):1–33.
8. King LS, Meehan MC. A history of the autopsy: a review. Am J Pathol. 1973;73(2):514–44.
9. Williams AN, Williams J. 'Proper to the duty of a Chirurgeon': Ambroise Paré and sixteenth century paediatric surgery. J Royal Soc Med. 2004;97:446–9.
10. The Workes of That Famous Chirurgion Ambroise Parey, 1649 English Translation; Accessible at: https://archive.org/stream/workesofthatfamo00par?ref=ol#page/n0/mode/2up.
11. Hamby WB. The case reports and autopsy records of Ambroise Paré. Springfield: C.C. Thomas Publisher; 1960.
12. Emmert JM. State medicine, past, present and future. JAMA. 1902;38(24):1568–78.
13. Smith S. Development of Forensic Medicine. J Pub Law. 1954;3:304–18.
14. Duffin J. Questioning medicine in the seventeenth-century Rome: the consultations of Paolo Zacchia. Can Bull Med Hist. 2011;28(1):149–70.
15. Foster B. The history of medicine and of the medical profession. Northwestern Lancet. 1898;18:261–6.
16. Brittain RP. The history of legal medicine: Charlemagne. Medico-Legal J. 1966;34:122–3.
17. Gerber SR. Expert medical testimony and the medical expert. Case Western Law Review. 1954;5(2):174–91.
18. Brittain RP. Origins of legal medicine: the origins of legal medicine in France. Medico-Legal J. 1966;34(3):168–74.
19. Brittain RP. Origins of legal medicine: Constitutio Criminalis Carolina. Medico-Legal J. 1965;33(3):124–7.
20. Brittain RP. Origins of legal medicine: the origins of legal medicine in France: Henri IV and Louis XIV. Medico-Legal J. 1967;35:25–8.
21. Cecchetto G, Bajanowski T, Cecci R, Favretto D, Graherr S, et al. Back to the future – part 1. The medico-legal autopsy from ancient civilization to the post-genomic era. Int J Legal Med. 2017;131:1069–83.
22. Hansma P. The evolution of the autopsy. Acad For Pathol. 2015;5(4):638–49.
23. Leidinger B, Lee WR. Marschalck, enforced convergence: political change and cause-of-death registration in the Hansestadt Bremen, 1860-1914. Contin Chang. 1997;12(2):221–46.
24. Madea B, editor. History of forensic medicine. Bonn: Lehmanns Media; 2017.
25. Reese DM. Fundamentals—Rudolf Virchow and modern medicine. West J Med. 1998;169(2):105–8.
26. Silver GA. Virchow, the heroic model in medicine: health policy by accolade. Am J Pub Hlth. 1986;77(1):82–8.
27. Chaille SE. Origin and progress of medical jurisprudence 1776-1876. J Crim Law and Criminol. 1949;40(4):397–444.
28. Forbes TR. Surgeons at the Bailey: English forensic medicine to 1878. New Haven: Yale University; 1985.

29. Eckert W. The development of forensic medicine in the United Kingdom from the 18th century. Am J For Med Pathol. 1992;13(2):124–31.
30. Wecht CH. The history of legal medicine. J Am Acad Psych Law. 2005;33(2):245–51.
31. Eckert J. New exhibit highlights Harvard's history with legal medicine, Center for the History of Medicine Center News. Accessible at: https://cms.www.countway.harvard.edu/wp/?tag=department-of-legal-medicine.
32. Watson KD. Forensic medicine in western society. New York: Routledge; 2011.
33. Butler SM. Forensic medicine and death investigation in medieval England. New York: Routledge; 2015.
34. Hunnisett J. The medieval coroner. Cambridge: Cambridge Univ Press; 1961.
35. Origins of the Coroner's Office, Univ of Georgia ehistory, CSI: Dixie webpage, 2014. Accessible at: https://csidixie.org/genesis/origins-coroners-office.
36. Wecht CH, Koehler SA. Death investigation systems: United States of America. In: Encyclopedia of forensic and legal medicine, vol. 2. Amsterdam: Elsevier; 2016. p. 42–50.
37. Loar C. Medical knowledge and the early modern English Coroner's inquest. Social Hist Med. 2010;23(3):475–91.
38. Dorries C. Coroners' courts: a guide to law and practice. 3d ed. Oxford: Oxford Univ Press; 2014.
39. Jentzen JM. Death investigation in America: coroners, medical examiners, and the pursuit of medical certainty. Cambridge: Harvard Univ Press; 2009.
40. Eckert WG. Medicolegal investigation in new York City: history and activities 1918-1978. Am J For Med Pathol. 1983;4(1):33–54.
41. LeBrun G. Call me if It's murder (It's time to tell). New York: Bantam; 1965.
42. Blum D. The Poisoner's handbook: murder and the birth of forensic medicine in Jazz age. New York: Penguin; 2011.
43. National Association of Medical Examiners(NAME). The history of the National Association of Medical Examiners, 2017 edition. Accessible at: https://www.dropbox.com/s/mlt4m8dqjf-pvz74/NAME%20e-book%202017%2011-24-17.pdf?dl=0.
44. Centers for Disease Control and Prevention (CDC). Death investigation systems webpage. Accessible at: https://www.cdc.gov/phlp/publications/coroner/death.html.
45. National Science and Technology Council, White House Office of Science and Technology Policy. Strengthening the medicolegal death investigation system: improving data systems, Sept 2016. Accessible at: https://obamawhitehouse.archives.gov/sites/default/files/microsites/ostp/NSTC/strengthening_the_medicolegal_death_investigation_system_final.pdf.
46. Hickman MJ, Hughes KA, Strom KJ, Ropero-Miller JD. Medical examiners and coroners' offices, 2004, NCJ 216756, Bureau of Justice Statistics, June 2007. Accessible at: https://www.bjs.gov/content/pub/pdf/meco04.pdf.
47. Hanzlick R, Combs D. Medical examiner and coroner systems: history and trends. JAMA. 1998;279(11):870–4.
48. National Vital Statistics System Homepage. Accessible at: https://www.cdc.gov/nchs/nvss/index.htm.
49. Web-based Injury Statistics Query and Reporting System (WISQARS) Homepage. Accessible at: https://www.cdc.gov/injury/wisqars/index.html.
50. National Violent Death Reporting System (NVDRS) Homepage: Accessible at: https://www.cdc.gov/violenceprevention/nvdrs/index.html.
51. Sudden Unexplained Infant Death Investigation (SUIDI) Reporting Form Homepage, Accessible at: https://www.cdc.gov/sids/suidrf.htm.
52. Strengthening Forensic Science in the United States: a path forward, 228091, National Academies Press, 2009, Available at: https://www.nap.edu/catalog/12589/strengthening-forensic-science-in-the-united-states-a-path-forward.
53. Ubelaker DH, editor. The global practice of forensic science. Hoboken: Wiley-Blackwell; 2015.

54. American Board of Medicolegal Death Investigation (ABMDI) homepage. Accessible at: http://www.abmdi.org/.
55. National Association of Medical Examiners (NAME) Forensic Autopsy Performance Standards. 2016. Accessible at: https://name.memberclicks.net/assets/docs/684b2442-ae68-4e64-9ecc-015f8d0f849e.pdf.
56. National Association of Medical Examiners (NAME) Inspection and Accreditation webpage. Accessible at: https://name.memberclicks.net/assets/docs/03c15f65-4b30-4dce-af50-1583d2d1a203.pdf
57. Hanzlick R. Cause of death and the death certificate. Chicago: College of American Pathologists; 2006.
58. National Association of Medical Examiners (NAME) Death Certification webpage. Accessible at: https://www.thename.org/index.php?option=com_content&view=article&id=47:death-certification&catid=20:site-content&Itemid=151.
59. National Crime Information Center (NCIC) homepage. Accessible at: https://www.fbi.gov/services/cjis/ncic.
60. National Missing and Unidentified Persons System (NamUS) homepage, Accessible at: https://namus.gov/.
61. Van Ryn D, Van Ryn S, Cerak N, Cerak C, Cerak W, Tabb M. Mistaken identity: two families, one survivor, unwavering hope. New York: Simon & Schuster; 2009.
62. Office of the Assistant Secretary for Preparedness and Response (ASPR) webpage. Accessible at: https://www.phe.gov/about/aspr/pages/default.aspx.
63. Office of the Assistant Secretary for Preparedness and Response (ASPR) Disaster Mortuary Operational Response Teams (DMORT) webpage. Accessible at: https://www.phe.gov/Preparedness/responders/ndms/ndms-teams/Pages/dmort.aspx.
64. National Association of Medical Examiners (NAME). Standard operating procedures for mass fatality management. 2010. https://www.thename.org/assets/docs/31434c24-8be0-4d2c-942a-8afde79ec1e7.pdf.
65. National Institute of Standards and Technology (NIST) Organization of Scientific Area Committees for Forensic Science (OSAC) Disaster Victim Identification Subcommittee webpage. Accessible at: https://www.nist.gov/topics/forensic-science/organization-scientific-area-committees-osac/disaster-victim-identification.
66. American Academy of Forensic Sciences (AAFS) Academy Standards Board (ASB) Consensus Bodies webpage. Accessible at: https://asb.aafs.org/consensus-bodies/.
67. *The Pathologist in Court*, College of Pathologists, 2003. Accessible as an ebook at: http://wdn2.ipublishcentral.com/college_american_pathologists/viewinside/500034861276787.
68. Weinberg M, Weedn VW, Weinberg S, Fowler D. Characteristics of medical examiner/coroner offices accredited by the National Association of medical examiners. J For Sci. 2013;58(5):1193–9.
69. Final Draft Views on Increasing the Number, Retention, and Quality of Board-Certified Forensic Pathologists, National Commission on Forensic Science (NCFS). Accessible at: https://www.justice.gov/archives/ncfs/medicolegal-death-investigation.
70. National Commission on Forensic Sciences archived website. Accessible at: https://www.justice.gov/archives/ncfs.
71. Weedn VW. Recent developments in the forensic sciences, United States Attorneys'. Bulletin 2017;65(1):3–10. Accessible at: https://www.justice.gov/usao/resources/united-states-attorneys-bulletins.
72. Organization of Scientific Area Committees website. Accessible at: https://swgmdi.org/.
73. Scientific Working Group on Medicolegal Death Investigation website. Accessible at: http://swgmdi.org/images/si4.fpsupplyreportpublisheddecember2012.pdf 21.
74. Strengthening the Medicolegal Death Investigation System: Accreditation and Certification, Office of Science and Technology Policy, Dec 2016. Accessible at: http://www.thecfso.org/advocacy/2017/OSTP_accreditation_recommendation.pdf.

75. Consortium of Forensic Science Organizations (CFSO) Homepage. Accessible at: http://www.thecfso.org/.
76. Final Draft Recommendation on Formation of a National Office of Medicolegal Death Investigation, National Commission on Forensic Science (NCFS). Accessible at: https://www.justice.gov/archives/ncfs/medicolegal-death-investigation.
77. National Institute of Justice (NIJ) Coverdell National Forensic Science Improvements Grants Program homepage. Accessible at: https://www.nij.gov/topics/forensics/lab-operations/capacity/nfsia/pages/welcome.aspx.
78. Hanzlick RL. A synoptic review of the 1954 model postmortem examinations act. Acad For Pathol. 2014;4(4):451–4.
79. Weedn VW. Model medical examiner legislation. Acad For Pathol. 2015;5(4):614–7.
80. Final Draft Recommendation on Model Legislation for Medicolegal Death Investigation Systems, National Commission on Forensic Science (NCFS). Accessible at: https://www.justice.gov/archives/ncfs/medicolegal-death-investigation.
81. Weiss D, McLeod-Henning, Waltke H. Using advanced imaging technologies to enhance autopsy practices. NIJ J. 2017;270. Accessible at: https://www.nij.gov/journals/279/Pages/using-advanced-imaging-technologies-to-enhance-autopsy.aspx.
82. Grabherr S, Baumann P, Minoiu C, Fahrni S, Mangin P. Post-mortem imaging in forensic investigations: current utility, limitations, and ongoing developments. Res Rep For Med Sci. 2016;6:25–37.
83. Villa C, Olsen KB, Hansen SH. Virtual animation of victim-specific 3D models obtained from CT scans for forensic reconstructions: living and dead subjects. For Sci Int. 2017;278:e27–33.

Part IV

The Autopsy as a Tool of Discovery

The Science of Rapid Research Autopsy

8

Jun Fan and Christine A. Iacobuzio-Donahue

Introduction

An autopsy is a medical procedure performed on a deceased person to determine the cause of death, among other purposes. While this procedure has been performed for centuries [1], the performance of an autopsy for the primary goal of collecting tissues to support basic and translational research is a much more contemporary concept. Research autopsies were first performed for the collection of brains to study neurological and psychiatric disease more than 200 years ago [2]. A more systematic approach to brain banking was initiated in the latter half of the twentieth century, which transitioned from only collecting examples of rare or particularly informative diseases to a systematic collection of all brains from consenting individuals that are fixed and sectioned using universally standardized protocols [2]. The utility of brain banks cannot be overstated, as they served as the grounds for discovery of the biochemical basis of Alzheimer's disease [3] and Parkinson's disease [4], among others. A recent and powerful example of the importance of brain banks is the description of chronic traumatic encephalopathy (CTE) in former athletes [5].

Given the success of brain banks for understanding neurologic disease, this approach has been applied to another important form of disease – cancer. Prostate cancer was the first tumor type to which the research autopsy was applied [6], with the terms "rapid" or "warm" autopsy used to reflect the reduced time to collection of tissues after death, as compared to clinical autopsies where 24 or more hours may

J. Fan
Department of Pathology, Stony Brook Medicine, Stony Brook, NY, USA
e-mail: Jun.fan@stonybrookmedicine.edu

C. A. Iacobuzio-Donahue (✉)
Department of Pathology, David M. Rubenstein Center for Pancreatic Cancer Research, Human Oncology and Pathogenesis Program, Memorial Sloan Kettering Cancer Center, New York, NY, USA
e-mail: iacobuzc@mskcc.org

J. E. Hooper, A. K. Williamson (eds.), *Autopsy in the 21st Century*,
https://doi.org/10.1007/978-3-319-98373-8_8

lapse between death and examination of the refrigerated body. Subsequently, research autopsies have been used to study a variety of tumor types with a profound influence on our understanding of the lethal cancer phenotype [7–11]. In this chapter, we aim to discuss the types of science that have been and can be supported by research autopsies, drawing from our own experience and that of the literature.

Quality of Rapid Research Autopsy Tissues

The word "postmortem" perpetuates a number of misconceptions about the quality and utility of tissues obtained after death for research [12, 13]. However, in autopsy pathology degraded tissue is the norm, and this field has made numerous technical advances despite this perceived obstacle [14]. When one considers that rapid research autopsies represent the "best of the best" tissue quality in autopsy pathology, it becomes clearer that postmortem tissue can be of tremendous value in basic and translational research. Table 8.1 illustrates the benefits of research autopsy tissues compared to other forms of banked tissue.

Perimortem Factors Influencing Tissue Quality

Unlike in the forensic setting where deceased individuals may be exposed to the outside elements of excessive heat, cold, moisture, and/or animal activity [15], patients who participate in research autopsies die in less variable settings, i.e., home,

Table 8.1 Tissue characteristics from rapid research autopsy samples vs other sources

	Rapid autopsy	Surgery	Core biopsy
Sample amounts obtained	Unlimited	Limited	Very limited
Lesional representation	High	Questionable	Questionable
Quality of DNA	Well-preserved	Well-preserved	Well-preserved
Quality of RNA	Perimortem factors, PMI, and tissue type dependent	Usually high, can be tissue type dependent	Usually high, can be tissue type dependent
Quality of protein	Generally high (dependent on analyte)	Generally high (dependent on analyte)	Generally high (dependent on analyte)
Normal/diseased matched samples	Yes	Maybe	No
Longitudinal sampling	No (end point)	Potentially	Potentially
Spatial sampling	Yes	Potentially	No
Multiorgan sampling	Yes	No	No
Immortalization of tumor	Yes	Yes	Yes

hospice, or the hospital [16]. Thus, extreme elements are relatively insignificant compared to the perimortem and postmortem intervals themselves.

After death, the core body temperature cools at an approximate rate of 1.5 °F until reaching room temperature [15]. During this time, tissues are still present in the body but are not being perfused, an interval known as "warm ischemia." By contrast, "cold ischemia" refers to the time after tissues are removed from the body until they are stabilized by flash freezing or fixation in formalin [17]. For research autopsies, warm ischemia accounts for the majority of the postmortem interval [16, 18]. In the rare event of extremely short postmortem intervals (1–2 h) [19], warm ischemia still remains the longest interval as tissues can be removed and stabilized within minutes of opening the body cavity. Thus, in aggregate cold ischemia is far less damaging to the molecular features of the samples than warm ischemia [17, 19]. Nonetheless, in both warm and cold ischemia, the extent of changes in specific molecules cannot be reliably predicted without formal investigation [19–22]. Equally as important to the postmortem interval is the mode of death of a patient. For example, patients who experienced a prolonged agonal state, such as due to sepsis or multiorgan failure, have lesser tissue quality than those who die of more sudden causes, for example, a thromboembolic event [23, 24]. Thus, molecular damage that occurs due to warm ischemia can occur even before death in hypoperfused organs and soft tissues of the extremities.

Deoxyribonucleic Acid (DNA)

Among nucleic acids, the most information regarding stability in different environments exists for DNA. DNA is intrinsically highly stable by nature of its hydrogen bonds within the double-stranded helix, particularly between guanine and cytosine pairs [25]. Nonetheless DNA has been shown to undergo hydrolytic DNA damage at a predictable rate, thereby serving as a sensor of DNA quality [26, 27]. We have previously performed a quantitative analysis of DNA quality in a range of normal tissues from patients who underwent a research autopsy and found that high-quality DNA was present in 89% of samples analyzed including in those in which RNA quality was poor [20]. High postmortem DNA stabilities have also been observed in other studies of human specimens from the brain, lymph nodes, and skeletal muscle [24, 28]. In our experience, DNA degradation can be compensated for by use of a different normal tissue from the same patient (most common approach) or by extraction of a larger amount of the degraded tissue to increase the net yield of high-quality DNA for downstream analyses.

Ribonucleic Acid (RNA)

Unlike DNA, RNA is highly sensitive to the peri- and postmortem interval in a tissue-specific manner [20, 29, 30]. Metrics of RNA quality commonly rely on the RNA integrity number, or RIN, using an Agilent Bioanalyzer system. With this system, an RIN value of 10 implies no RNA degradation, and 0 implies complete degradation. However, because this metric is based on ribosomal RNA, it is a surrogate assessment of messenger RNA quality. We and others have used the RIN value to evaluate RNA quality in normal and diseased cancer tissues from research autopsy participants [20, 29, 30]. RIN values showed an expected inverse correlation with postmortem interval in most tissues. However, outliers to this pattern appear to be the heart and skeletal muscle; even at 36 or more hours after death, we found the median RIN values for these tissues were 7.9 and 8.8, respectively. Somewhat unexpectedly, the kidney had the lowest quality with a median RIN of only 6.2 in cases with postmortem intervals of 4 h or less. Using normal pancreas and pancreatic cancer tissues from the same patient, we also determined if postmortem intervals affect cancer tissue RNA quality to the same extent as normal tissues. This was not the case, with cancer tissues having greater abundance and higher RIN values than their matched normal pancreas. Thus, across patients and even within a single patient, independent studies indicate the RIN value of one tissue is not predictive of RIN values in other tissues within a given postmortem interval [20, 30].

Gupta et al. performed a more objective study of global gene expression using hearts from research autopsy participants for cancer (non-failed hearts) and cardiac explants (failed hearts) subjected to 24 h of cold ischemia [31]. The 24-h autopsy simulation was designed to reflect a typical autopsy scenario where a body may begin cooling to ambient temperature for approximately 12 h, before transportation and storage in a refrigerated room in a morgue. Overall, less than 2.5% of genes, largely belonging to immune response and energy metabolism-related processes, showed fluctuations in expression over the 24-h period. Furthermore, RNA expression was reproducible over 24 h of autolysis with 95% genes showing less than a 1.2-fold change. The authors concluded that RNA from autopsy-derived tissue, even with up to 24 h of autolysis, could be used to identify biologically relevant expression pattern differences, thus serving as a practical source for gene expression experiments. While heart tissue appears to have greater stability than other tissues for RNA in general, such studies are informative for the extent of change that can be expected in the postmortem setting when analyzing complex datasets.

Protein

Proteins represent a diverse array of biomolecules with varying isoforms from the same RNA transcript and one or more posttranslational modifications that act to change the stability of the protein or alter its subcellular location. In one of the few studies to assess changes to the proteome during cold ischemia using mass spectrometry, 30% of peaks were found to change greater than twofold within 30 min of removal of the tissue from the body; most changes occurred within 15 min [32]. While this finding does not address if these changes are biologically meaningful or if the 30% of peaks corresponded to a particular class of peptides, it does indicate that the steady-state levels of some proteins may be perturbed soon after devascularization.

Phosphoproteins are particularly tenuous in general, with half-lives on the order of minutes in controlled studies [33]. In a study to determine the effects of cold ischemia on the proteome, specimens of the intestine and liver were studied by reverse protein phase arrays (RPPA) using a variety of antibodies including many against phosphoproteins [34]. The vast majority of proteins remained unchanged in abundance from 30 min to 360 min, and interpatient variability was much greater than intrapatient variability in abundance. Finally, the authors concluded that changes during warm ischemia were much more extensive than those caused during 30 min of cold ischemia, again illustrating the significance of perimortem factors in biomolecule quality.

A separate and independent immunohistochemical study of 18 targets (metalloproteinases and their inhibitors, scavenge receptors, and two forms of glycation end products) in normal tissues collected during the postmortem interval showed analogous results [22]. The authors studied 16 different normal tissues to evaluate 48 h of autolysis in a warm or cold environment. No systematic diminution of signal intensity, confirmed by digital analysis or Western blotting, was observed during the initial period of 24 h indicating these classes of proteins degrade slowly and faithfully maintain their immunohistochemical characteristics in devitalized tissues.

Immortalization of Cancer Tissues

While the definition of death itself may range depending on ethical, legal, or medical circumstances [35], some cellular processes continue after cardiorespiratory arrest occurs [36]. This is perhaps best illustrated by the ability to create immortalized models from postmortem tissues, specifically cancer tissues. Tumor types that have been successfully xenografted or cultured from postmortem tissues include prostate cancer, pancreatic cancer, breast cancer, and pediatric brain and soft tissue tumors [6, 18, 37–40]. Organized and objective studies of the features of postmortem tissues that best support creation of such models are uncommon. However, Embuscado et al. reported engraftment rates of 57% when using samples of pancreatic cancer collected within 6 h of death, one $CD1^{nu/nu}$ mouse per tumor and two sites of implantation per mouse [18]. In the same study, the authors noted that metastases were more likely to engraft than primary tumors from the same patient. By contrast, Rubin et al. reported a 5% engraftment rate from metastatic prostate cancer samples despite very short postmortem intervals and exceptional care to implant viable samples without necrosis [6]. Collectively these findings indicate inherent biologic differences within a tumor type and between tumor types contribute to the ability to establish patient-derived xenograft models from research autopsy participants beyond the postmortem interval. More recent efforts have centered on the creation of patient-derived organoid models that are thought to more closely recapitulate patient biology, with reported success in generating organoid cultures from ovarian cancer and colon cancers collected postmortem [38].

Science Supported by Rapid Research Autopsy Tissues

Given the stability of DNA, whole exome and whole genome studies that utilize postmortem tissue are the most numerous types of analysis reported thus far. Pancreatic cancer, prostate cancer, and breast cancer are the three tumor types that account for the majority of these studies, likely because rapid autopsy programs related to these tumor types have been in operation the longest. However, the below approaches can be and/or have been applied to any tumor type or disease for which postmortem tissues are available [41, 42]. In addition to the below discussion, a summary of the methods that have been proven to work, are expected to work (provided efforts are made to optimize conditions for these postmortem tissues) or have not been tested using rapid research autopsy tissues as shown in Fig. 8.1.

Gene Discovery

The quality of DNA in postmortem tissues illustrates their utility in sequencing studies. In prostate cancer, research autopsy tissues from men who died of their disease were used to identify the *CDKN1B* and *ETV6* genes on chromosome 12p as targets of homozygous deletion [43]. Jones et al. [44] used 24 pancreatic cancers, 7 of which were xenografts or cell lines established from research autopsy participants, to provide the first characterization of the pancreatic cancer exome. Interestingly, there was no difference in the total mutational burden or enrichment for any specific gene or pathway among the autopsy-derived samples and the surgically derived samples.

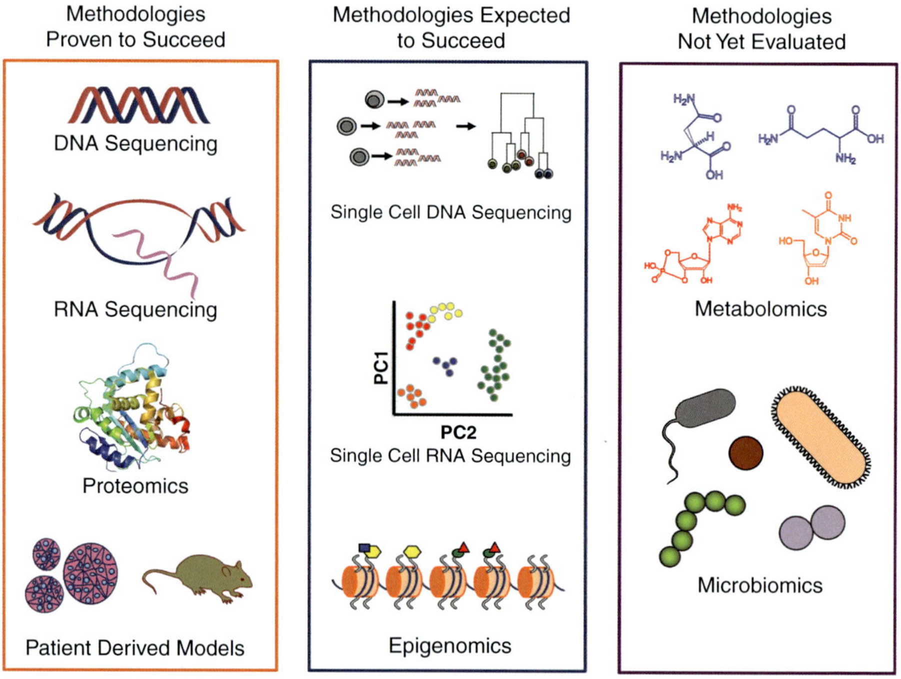

Fig. 8.1 Research methodologies that can be supported by rapid research autopsy tissue resources

Characterizations and Timing of Subclonal Evolution

A particular strength of research autopsies over other methods of tissue collection is that all samples from the patient are accessible for banking and downstream studies. Such sample sets greatly facilitate studies of genetic heterogeneity in a single patient or across cohorts of similarly treated patients and have been used for this purpose in a variety of tumor types (Fig. 8.2). In breast cancers, WES and copy

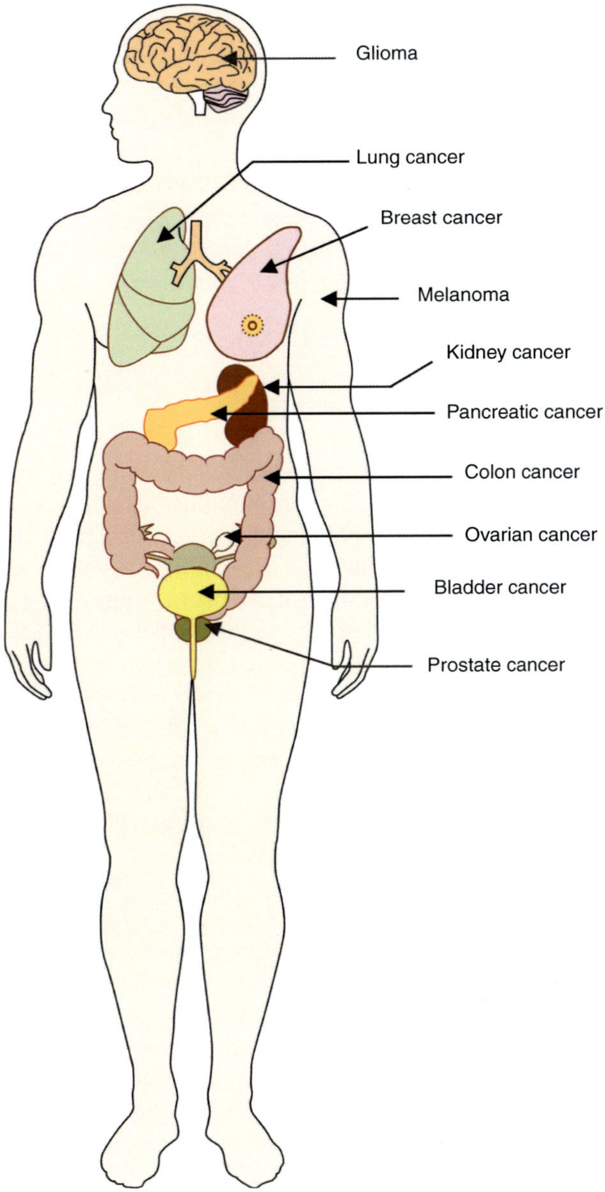

Fig. 8.2 Tumor types that have been characterized by next-generation sequencing using rapid research autopsy samples

number analyses (CNAs) of matched primary and metastatic tumors from ten autopsied patients revealed two modes of disease progression, one in which all metastases descend from a common precursor and a second in which the multiple metastases are seeded from different precursor cells present in the primary tumor [45]. In metastatic prostate cancers, CNAs revealed that most metastatic prostate cancers have monoclonal origins despite common genetic heterogeneity of the primary tumors [11]. Furthermore, Gundem et al. found that metastasis to metastasis spread was common in metastatic prostate cancer through de novo seeding of tertiary metastases or transfer of multiple tumor clones between metastatic sites [46]. In metastatic pancreatic cancers, Campbell et al. [47] showed by massively parallel paired-end sequencing that the majority of structural rearrangements within the pancreatic cancer genome were shared among the primary tumor and metastases, indicating that they occurred before the development of metastatic disease. Similar findings using WES of an overlapping subset of samples were reported by Yachida et al. as well [48]. Through genomic profiling of a patient with lung cancer who exhibited an exceptional response to ERBB2-directed therapies, Biswas et al. found profound genomic heterogeneity and patterns consistent with early metastasis from the primary tumor site with parallel independent evolution in the draining lymph nodes [42].

Computational Modeling

The extent of metadata provided by research autopsies has spurred computational studies to deconvolute patterns not otherwise appreciable. Using breast cancer tissues collected from rapid autopsy cases, Almendro et al. [10] calculated Shannon indices of intratumoral diversity within phenotypically distinct cell populations and found that the treatment-naïve primary tumor and lymph node metastases were genetically diverse compared to the metastases that were more divergent. Yachida et al. [48] relied on data generated from whole exome sequencing of seven metastases to generate a computational model estimating the timeline for pancreatic cancer from its initiation from a normal cell until the time that is has disseminated to distant organs. Makohon-Moore et al. [49] created a computational model of expected genetic heterogeneity among normal cells in a single organ and applied this model to data generated from Stage IV treatment-naïve pancreatic cancers, thereby providing the first quantitative estimates of genetic heterogeneity in metastasis-initiating cells.

Computational modeling of treatment dynamics using rapid autopsy resources has similarly proven useful. Haeno et al. used the timing of primary and metastasis growth patterns across a large cohort of research autopsy patients to determine by computational models the optimal timing and mode of treatment for resected pancreatic cancers [50]. A similar approach was utilized in breast cancers that indicated a lower degree of genetic diversity pretreatment was associated with an improved outcome, and this data formed the basis for a computational model incorporating single cell genotypes and phenotypes to predict tumor evolution [51].

DNA Methylation

Just as sequencing has proven insightful to the dynamics of metastasis, studies reliant on DNA methylation have also been successfully applied to tissues from rapid autopsy participants. Among the first study to do so was in autopsied breast cancer patients for which methylation of multiple gene promoters was assessed in different metastatic sites, revealing that promoter hypermethylation for genes important for breast cancer biology such as *RASSF1a*, *HIN1*, *cyclin D2*, *Twist*, *estrogen receptor* α, *APC1*, or *RAR*β remained unchanged during progression from primary to metastatic disease [8]. Using genome-scale analyses of DNA methylation in metastatic prostate cancer samples, Aryee et al. found a similar pattern in that DNA hypermethylation patterns were highly concordant among the samples from any one individual but variable across patients [52]. Subsequently, rapid autopsy tissues were used to further demonstrate that DNA hypomethylation occurs later than DNA hypermethylation and is heterogeneous across metastatic sites [53].

Gene Expression

Despite some degree of degradation, RNA can be evaluated at a global level from postmortem tissues. Campagna et al. [54] used gene expression microarrays to study matched primary and metastatic pancreatic cancers from a variety of tumor sites. They identified significant differences in expression in association with growth at the primary site that were most prominent in genes associated with MAPK and Wnt pathway, metabolism, immune regulation, and cell-cell and cell-matrix interactions within the infiltrating carcinoma. Likewise, Gupta et al. [31] used expression microarrays to demonstrate that postmortem cardiac tissues maintain their expression profiles despite prolonged warm or cold ischemia. Fan et al. [20] used RNA-sequencing to analyze five matched pairs of normal pancreas and pancreatic cancer tissue from research autopsy participants, all with RIN values >5.0. Sequencing libraries showed a sound distribution of coverage across transcripts and fragment lengths that were irrespective of RIN value, and genes overrepresented in normal pancreas or pancreatic cancer were consistent with known biomarkers and tissue homeostasis. Moreover, two recurrent fusions were identified in six samples. Using a larger scope of tumor types and more comprehensive analyses, Pisapia et al. [38] also found that RNA-sequencing quality from postmortem tissues was robust and identified potentially meaningful alterations that included novel gene fusion candidates such as *ZNF526-MEGF8*.

Human Proteome

A triumph of research autopsies is their support of the first reported characterization of the human proteome [55]. Using high-resolution Fourier-transform mass spectrometry, Kim et al. performed an in-depth proteomic profiling of 17 different adult human tissues, all from research autopsy participants. Normal tissues from at least three patients were used for analysis to account for interpatient variability. They identified the proteins encoded by 17,294 genes accounting for approximately 84% of the total annotated protein-coding genes in humans. Data of this project is freely available as an interactive web-based resource at http://www.humanproteomemap.org.

Models of Rare Diseases

For several tumor types, premortem diagnostic tissue specimens are not available.

This may be because the tumor type itself is very rare or biopsy cannot be performed without putting the patient at significant risk. Thus, the creation of model systems from research autopsies has proven useful in the ability to obtain tissue for the creation of patient-derived xenografts, organoids, or cell culture models. Yachida et al. [56] described the autopsy of a patient with primary small cell carcinoma of the pancreas and the creation of a cell line, A99, from this tumor. Cell lines and xenografts of diffuse intrinsic pontine gliomas (DIPG) of children have been established [57, 58], thereby providing a critical resource for understanding this rare and lethal tumor type. A similarly successful approach has been to establish a xenograft model of embryonal rhabdomyosarcoma [59]. While this is one of the most common soft tissue tumor types in children, overall it is a rare tumor type with few therapeutic options once recurrent disease occurs [60].

Future Directions in the Science of Rapid Research Autopsy

As stated in our introduction, an autopsy is a medical procedure performed on a deceased patient to determine the cause of death, among other purposes. However, with advances in medical technology and imaging, the postmortem examination has declined dramatically [61]. Given that postmortem tissues are amenable to the same methodologies and technologies that have formed the basis for personalized medicine, a comprehensive and integrated analysis of various levels of -omic data has the potential to uncover genotype-phenotype relationships not yet appreciated, ultimately poising autopsies to once again provide the final determinations of disease-related physiology (Fig. 8.3). This possibility is buttressed by reports in a variety of tumor types where integrated clinical, next-generation sequencing and transcriptome analyses of multi-sampled end-stage cancers from rapid research autopsy participants are performed. For each patient these studies offered potential mechanisms of resistance and provide insight into tumor type specific dynamics not otherwise appreciated by any other approach [38, 41, 62].

The ability to collect both normal and diseased tissues from a single patient, and from many patients, opens the door to the development of powerful methods of data integration for understanding human health, development, aging, and disease on an unprecedented scale [63]. These include system genomics approaches that can

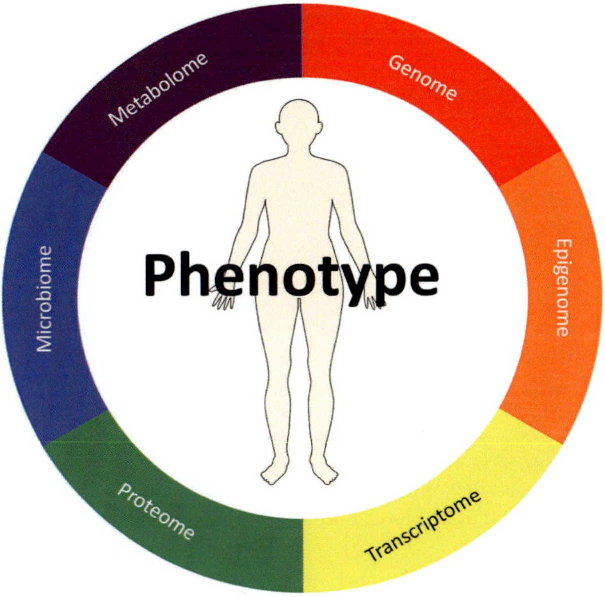

Fig. 8.3 Proposed utility of postmortem examination in the future

unravel the complexities and relative contributions of a large number of variables across multiple levels of biologic regulation, i.e., metabolism, DNA damage, inflammation, and epigenome regulation, not possible from any single data type [63]. Such approaches should take into account peri- and postmortem variables as well, thus allowing a separation of the biology of death itself from the disease of interest, and may require multi-institutional and/or multi-national collaborations for success, similar to that achieved by The Cancer Genome Atlas (https://cancergenome.nih.gov).

References

1. Connolly AJ, Finkbeiner WE, Ursell PC, Davis RL. Autopsy pathology: a manual and atlas. Elsevier Health Sciences; 2015. Philadelphia, PA: USA.
2. Kretzschmar H. Brain banking: opportunities, challenges and meaning for the future. Nat Rev Neurosci. 2009;10(1):70–8. Nature Publishing Group.
3. Glenner GG, Wong CW. Alzheimer's disease: initial report of the purification and characterization of a novel cerebrovascular amyloid protein. Biochem Biophys Res Commun. 1984;120(3):885–90.
4. Spillantini MG, Crowther RA, Jakes R, Hasegawa M, Goedert M. Alpha-Synuclein in filamentous inclusions of Lewy bodies from Parkinson's disease and dementia with lewy bodies. Proc Natl Acad Sci U S A. 1998;95(11):6469–73. PMCID: PMC27806. National Academy of Sciences.
5. Mez J, Daneshvar DH, Kiernan PT, Abdolmohammadi B, Alvarez VE, Huber BR, Alosco ML, Solomon TM, Nowinski CJ, McHale L, Cormier KA, Kubilus CA, Martin BM, Murphy L, Baugh CM, Montenigro PH, Chaisson CE, Tripodis Y, Kowall NW, Weuve J, McClean MD, Cantu RC, Goldstein LE, Katz DI, Stern RA, Stein TD, McKee AC. Clinicopathological evaluation of chronic traumatic encephalopathy in players of American football. JAMA. 2017;318(4):360–70. PMCID: PMC5807097.

6. Rubin MA, Putzi M, Mucci N, Smith DC, Wojno K, Korenchuk S, Pienta KJ. Rapid ("warm") autopsy study for procurement of metastatic prostate cancer. Clin Cancer Res. 2000;6(3):1038–45.
7. Iacobuzio-Donahue CA, Fu B, Yachida S, Luo M, Abe H, Henderson CM, Vilardell F, Wang Z, Keller JW, Banerjee P, Herman JM, Cameron JL, Yeo CJ, Halushka MK, Eshleman JR, Raben M, Klein AP, Hruban RH, Hidalgo M, Laheru D. DPC4 gene status of the primary carcinoma correlates with patterns of failure in patients with pancreatic cancer. J Clin Oncol. 2009;27(11):1806–13. PMCID: PMC2668706.
8. Wu JM, Fackler MJ, Halushka MK, Molavi DW, Taylor ME, Teo WW, Griffin C, Fetting J, Davidson NE, De Marzo AM, Hicks JL, Chitale D, Ladanyi M, Sukumar S, Argani P. Heterogeneity of breast cancer metastases: comparison of therapeutic target expression and promoter methylation between primary tumors and their multifocal metastases. Clin Cancer Res. 2008;14(7):1938–46. PMCID: PMC2965068. American Association for Cancer Research.
9. Avigdor BE, Cimino-Mathews A, Demarzo AM, Hicks JL, Shin J, Sukumar S, Fetting J, Argani P, Park BH, Wheelan SJ. Mutational profiles of breast cancer metastases from a rapid autopsy series reveal multiple evolutionary trajectories. JCI Insight. 2017;2(24):1–10. PMCID: PMC5752302.
10. Almendro V, Kim HJ, Cheng Y-K, Gönen M, Itzkovitz S, Argani P, van Oudenaarden A, Sukumar S, Michor F, Polyak K. Genetic and phenotypic diversity in breast tumor metastases. Cancer Res. 2014;74(5):1338–48. PMCID: PMC3963810. American Association for Cancer Research.
11. Liu W, Laitinen S, Khan S, Vihinen M, Kowalski J, Yu G, Chen L, Ewing CM, Eisenberger MA, Carducci MA, Nelson WG, Yegnasubramanian S, Luo J, Wang Y, Xu J, Isaacs WB, Visakorpi T, Bova GS. Copy number analysis indicates monoclonal origin of lethal metastatic prostate cancer. Nat Med. 2009;15(5):559–65. PMCID: PMC2839160. Nature Publishing Group.
12. Quinn GP, Murphy D, Pratt C, Muñoz-Antonia T, Guerra L, Schabath MB, Leon ME, Haura E. Altruism in terminal cancer patients and rapid tissue donation program: does the theory apply? Med Health Care Philos. 2013;16(4):857–64. PMCID: PMC3735793.
13. Quinn GP, Pentz RD, Muñoz-Antonia T, Boyle TA, Schabath MB, Pratt CL, Shaffer A, Duarte LF, Bowman-Curci M, Antonia SJ, Chiappori AA, Creelan BC, Gray JE, Williams CC, Haura EB. Patient, caregiver and physician perspectives on participating in a thoracic rapid tissue donation program. Patient Educ Couns. 2018;101(4):703–10.
14. Sijen T. Molecular approaches for forensic cell type identification: on mRNA, miRNA, DNA methylation and microbial markers. Forensic Sci Int Genet. 2015;18:21–32.
15. Dolinak D, Matshes E, Lew EO. Forensic pathology: Elsevier; 2005. Burlington, MA: USA.
16. Alsop K, Thorne H, Sandhu S, Hamilton A, Mintoff C, Christie E, Spruyt O, Williams S, McNally O, Mileshkin L, Ananda S, Hallo J, Loi S, Scott C, Savas P, Devereux L, O'Brien P, Gunawardena S, Hampson C, Strachan K, Jaravaza RD, Francis V, Young G, Ranson D, Samaranayake R, Stevens D, Boyle S, Fedele C, Topp M, Ho G, Teo ZL, Taylor RA, Papargiris MM, Lawrence MG, Wang H, Risbridger GP, Haynes NM, Medon M, Johnstone RW, Vidacs E, Arnau GM, Vergara IA, Papenfuss AT, McArthur G, Waring P, Carvosso S, Angel C, Gyorki D, Solomon B, Mitchell G, et al. A community-based model of rapid autopsy in end-stage cancer patients. Nat Biotechnol. 2016;34(10):1010–4. Nature Publishing Group.
17. Atherton DS, Sexton KC, Otali D, Bell WC, Grizzle WE. Factors affecting the use of human tissues in biomedical research: implications in the design and operation of a biorepository. Methods Mol Biol. 2016;1381(Chapter 1):1–38. New York, NY: Springer New York.
18. Embuscado EE, Laheru D, Ricci F, Yun KJ, de Boom WS, Seigel A, Flickinger K, Hidalgo M, Bova GS, Iacobuzio-Donahue CA. Immortalizing the complexity of cancer metastasis: genetic features of lethal metastatic pancreatic cancer obtained from rapid autopsy. Cancer Biol Ther. 2005;4(5):548–54. PMCID: PMC2771924.
19. Grizzle WE, Otali D, Sexton KC, Atherton DS. Effects of cold ischemia on gene expression: a review and commentary. Biopreserv Biobank. 2016;14(6):548–58. PMCID: PMC5180081. Mary Ann Liebert, Inc. 140 Huguenot Street, 3rd Floor New Rochelle, NY 10801 USA.

20. Fan J, Khanin R, Sakamoto H, Zhong Y, Michael C, Pena D, Javier B, Wood LD, Iacobuzio-Donahue CA. Quantification of nucleic acid quality in postmortem tissues from a cancer research autopsy program. Oncotarget. 2016;7(41):66906–21. PMCID: PMC5341846. Impact Journals.
21. Halushka MK, Selvin E, Lu J, Macgregor AM, Cornish TC. Use of human vascular tissue microarrays for measurement of advanced glycation end products. J Histochem Cytochem. 2009;57(6):559–66. PMCID: PMC2690436. SAGE PublicationsSage CA: Los Angeles, CA.
22. Maleszewski J, Lu J, Fox-Talbot K, Halushka MK. Robust immunohistochemical staining of several classes of proteins in tissues subjected to autolysis. J Histochem Cytochem. 2007;55(6):597–606. SAGE Publications Sage CA: Los Angeles, CA.
23. Harrison PJ, Heath PR, Eastwood SL, Burnet PW, McDonald B, Pearson RC. The relative importance of premortem acidosis and postmortem interval for human brain gene expression studies: selective mRNA vulnerability and comparison with their encoded proteins. Neurosci Lett. 1995;200(3):151–4.
24. Bär W, Kratzer A, Mächler M, Schmid W. Postmortem stability of DNA. Forensic Sci Int. 1988;39(1):59–70.
25. Yakovchuk P, Protozanova E, Frank-Kamenetskii MD. Base-stacking and base-pairing contributions into thermal stability of the DNA double helix. Nucleic Acids Res. 2006;34(2):564–74. PMCID: PMC1360284.
26. Marrone A, Ballantyne J. Hydrolysis of DNA and its molecular components in the dry state. Forensic Sci Int Genet. 2010;4(3):168–77.
27. Allentoft ME, Collins M, Harker D, Haile J, Oskam CL, Hale ML, Campos PF, Samaniego JA, Gilbert MTP, Willerslev E, Zhang G, Scofield RP, Holdaway RN, Bunce M. The half-life of DNA in bone: measuring decay kinetics in 158 dated fossils. Proc Biol Sci. 2012;279(1748):4724–33. PMCID: PMC3497090. The Royal Society.
28. Hansen J, Lesnikova I, Funder AMD, Banner J. DNA and RNA analysis of blood and muscle from bodies with variable postmortem intervals. Forensic Sci Med Pathol. 2014;10(3):322–8. Springer US.
29. Birdsill AC, Walker DG, Lue L, Sue LI, Beach TG. Postmortem interval effect on RNA and gene expression in human brain tissue. Cell Tissue Bank. 2011;12(4):311–8. PMCID: PMC3343031. Springer Netherlands.
30. Walker DG, Whetzel AM, Serrano G, Sue LI, Lue L-F, Beach TG. Characterization of RNA isolated from eighteen different human tissues: results from a rapid human autopsy program. Cell Tissue Bank. 2016;17(3):361–75. PMCID: PMC5026224. Springer Netherlands.
31. Gupta S, Halushka MK, Hilton GM, Arking DE. Postmortem cardiac tissue maintains gene expression profile even after late harvesting. BMC Genomics. 2012;13(1):26. PMCID: PMC3342086. BioMed Central.
32. Spruessel A, Steimann G, Jung M, Lee SA, Carr T, Fentz A-K, Spangenberg J, Zornig C, Juhl HH, David KA. Tissue ischemia time affects gene and protein expression patterns within minutes following surgical tumor excision. BioTechniques. 2004;36(6):1030–7.
33. Espina V, Mueller C, Liotta LA. Phosphoprotein stability in clinical tissue and its relevance for reverse phase protein microarray technology. Methods Mol Biol. 2011;785(Chapter 3):23–43. PMCID: PMC3746012. Totowa, NJ: Humana Press.
34. Gündisch S, Hauck S, Sarioglu H, Schott C, Viertler C, Kap M, Schuster T, Reischauer B, Rosenberg R, Verhoef C, Mischinger H-J, Riegman P, Zatloukal K, Becker K-F. Variability of protein and phosphoprotein levels in clinical tissue specimens during the preanalytical phase. J Proteome Res. 2012;11(12):5748–62. American Chemical Society.
35. Schofield GM, Urch CE, Stebbing J, Giamas G. When does a human being die? QJM. 2015;108(8):605–9.
36. Pozhitkov AE, Noble PA. Gene expression in the twilight of death: the increase of thousands of transcripts has implications to transplantation, cancer, and forensic research. BioEssays. 2017;39(9):1700066.
37. Juric D, Castel P, Griffith M, Griffith OL, Won HH, Ellis H, Ebbesen SH, Ainscough BJ, Ramu A, Iyer G, Shah RH, Huynh T, Mino-Kenudson M, Sgroi D, Isakoff S, Thabet A, Elamine L,

Solit DB, Lowe SW, Quadt C, Peters M, Derti A, Schegel R, Huang A, Mardis ER, Berger MF, Baselga J, Scaltriti M. Convergent loss of PTEN leads to clinical resistance to a PI(3)Kα inhibitor. Nature. 2015;518(7538):240–4. PMCID: PMC4326538. Nature Publishing Group.
38. Pisapia DJ, Salvatore S, Pauli C, Hissong E, Eng K, Prandi D, Sailer V-W, Robinson BD, Park K, Cyrta J, Tagawa ST, Kossai M, Fontugne J, Kim R, Sigaras A, Rao R, Pancirer D, Faltas B, Bareja R, Molina AM, Nanus DM, Rajappa P, Souweidane MM, Greenfield J, Emde A-K, Robine N, Elemento O, Sboner A, Demichelis F, Beltran H, Rubin MA, Mosquera JM. Next-generation rapid autopsies enable tumor evolution tracking and generation of preclinical models. JCO Precis Oncol. 2017;2017. PMCID: PMC5761727. NIH Public Access. https://doi.org/10.1200/PO.16.00038. Epub 2017.
39. Meel MH, Sewing ACP, Waranecki P, Metselaar DS, Wedekind LE, Koster J, van Vuurden DG, Kaspers GJL, Hulleman E. Culture methods of diffuse intrinsic pontine glioma cells determine response to targeted therapies. Exp Cell Res. 2017;360(2):397–403.
40. Xie T, Musteanu M, Lopez-Casas PP, Shields DJ, Olson P, Rejto PA, Hidalgo M. Whole exome sequencing of rapid autopsy tumors and xenograft models reveals possible driver mutations underlying tumor progression. PLoS ONE. 2015;10(11):e0142631. Rooman I, editor. PMCID: PMC4640827. Public Library of Science.
41. Ascierto ML, Makohon-Moore A, Lipson EJ, Taube JM, McMiller TL, Berger AE, Fan J, Kaunitz G, Cottrell T, Kohutek Z, Favorov A, Makarov V, Riaz N, Chan TA, Cope L, Hruban RH, Pardoll DM, Taylor BS, Solit DB, Iacobuzio-Donahue CA, Topalian SL. Transcriptional mechanisms of resistance to anti-PD-1 therapy. Clin Cancer Res. 2017;23(12):3168–80. clincanres.0270.2016. PMCID: PMC5474192.
42. Biswas R, Gao S, Cultraro CM, Maity TK, Venugopalan A, Abdullaev Z, Shaytan AK, Carter CA, Thomas A, Rajan A, Song Y, Pitts S, Chen K, Bass S, Boland J, Hanada K-I, Chen J, Meltzer PS, Panchenko AR, Yang JC, Pack S, Giaccone G, Schrump DS, Khan J, Guha U. Genomic profiling of multiple sequentially acquired tumor metastatic sites from an "exceptional responder" lung adenocarcinoma patient reveals extensive genomic heterogeneity and novel somatic variants driving treatment response. Cold Spring Harb Mol Case Stud. 2016;2(6):a001263. PMCID: PMC5111000. Cold Spring Harbor Laboratory Press.
43. Kibel AS, Schutte M, Kern SE, Isaacs WB, Bova GS. Identification of 12p as a region of frequent deletion in advanced prostate cancer. Cancer Res. 1998;58(24):5652–5.
44. Jones S, Zhang X, Parsons DW, Lin JC-H, Leary RJ, Angenendt P, Mankoo P, Carter H, Kamiyama H, Jimeno A, Hong S-M, Fu B, Lin M-T, Calhoun ES, Kamiyama M, Walter K, Nikolskaya T, Nikolsky Y, Hartigan J, Smith DR, Hidalgo M, Leach SD, Klein AP, Jaffee EM, Goggins M, Maitra A, Iacobuzio-Donahue C, Eshleman JR, Kern SE, Hruban RH, Karchin R, Papadopoulos N, Parmigiani G, Vogelstein B, Velculescu VE, Kinzler KW. Core signaling pathways in human pancreatic cancers revealed by global genomic analyses. Science. 2008;321(5897):1801–6. PMCID: PMC2848990.
45. Brown D, Smeets D, Székely B, Larsimont D, Szász AM, Adnet P-Y, Rothé F, Rouas G, Nagy ZI, Faragó Z, Tőkés A-M, Dank M, Szentmártoni G, Udvarhelyi N, Zoppoli G, Pusztai L, Piccart M, Kulka J, Lambrechts D, Sotiriou C, Desmedt C. Phylogenetic analysis of metastatic progression in breast cancer using somatic mutations and copy number aberrations. Nat Commun. 2017;8:14944. PMCID: PMC5474888. Nature Publishing Group.
46. Gundem G, Van Loo P, Kremeyer B, Alexandrov LB, Tubio JMC, Papaemmanuil E, Brewer DS, Kallio HML, Högnäs G, Annala M, Kivinummi K, Goody V, Latimer C, O'Meara S, Dawson KJ, Isaacs W, Emmert-Buck MR, Nykter M, Foster C, Kote-Jarai Z, Easton D, Whitaker HC, ICGC Prostate Group, Neal DE, Cooper CS, Eeles RA, Visakorpi T, Campbell PJ, McDermott U, Wedge DC, Bova GS. The evolutionary history of lethal metastatic prostate cancer. Nature. 2015;520(7547):353–7. PMCID: PMC4413032. Nature Publishing Group.
47. Campbell PJ, Yachida S, Mudie LJ, Stephens PJ, Pleasance ED, Stebbings LA, Morsberger LA, Latimer C, McLaren S, Lin M-L, McBride DJ, Varela I, Nik-Zainal SA, Leroy C, Jia M, Menzies A, Butler AP, Teague JW, Griffin CA, Burton J, Swerdlow H, Quail MA, Stratton MR, Iacobuzio-Donahue C, Futreal PA. The patterns and dynamics of genomic instability in metastatic pancreatic cancer. Nature. 2010;467(7319):1109–13. PMCID: PMC3137369.

48. Yachida S, Jones S, Bozic I, Antal T, Leary R, Fu B, Kamiyama M, Hruban RH, Eshleman JR, Nowak MA, Velculescu VE, Kinzler KW, Vogelstein B, Iacobuzio-Donahue CA. Distant metastasis occurs late during the genetic evolution of pancreatic cancer. Nature. 2010;467(7319):1114–7. PMCID: PMC3148940. Nature Research.
49. Makohon-Moore AP, Zhang M, Reiter JG, Bozic I, Allen B, Kundu D, Chatterjee K, Wong F, Jiao Y, Kohutek ZA, Hong J, Attiyeh M, Javier B, Wood LD, Hruban RH, Nowak MA, Papadopoulos N, Kinzler KW, Vogelstein B, Iacobuzio-Donahue CA. Limited heterogeneity of known driver gene mutations among the metastases of individual patients with pancreatic cancer. Nat Genet. 2017;49(3):358–66. PMCID: PMC5663439. Nature Research.
50. Haeno H, Gonen M, Davis MB, Herman JM, Iacobuzio-Donahue CA, Michor F. Computational modeling of pancreatic cancer reveals kinetics of metastasis suggesting optimum treatment strategies. Cell. 2012;148(1–2):362–75. PMCID: PMC3289413.
51. Almendro V, Cheng Y-K, Randles A, Itzkovitz S, Marusyk A, Ametller E, Gonzalez-Farre X, Muñoz M, Russnes HG, Helland A, Rye IH, Børresen-Dale A-L, Maruyama R, van Oudenaarden A, Dowsett M, Jones RL, Reis-Filho J, Gascon P, Gönen M, Michor F, Polyak K. Inference of tumor evolution during chemotherapy by computational modeling and in situ analysis of genetic and phenotypic cellular diversity. Cell Rep. 2014;6(3):514–27. PMCID: PMC3928845.
52. Aryee MJ, Liu W, Engelmann JC, Nuhn P, Gurel M, Haffner MC, Esopi D, Irizarry RA, Getzenberg RH, Nelson WG, Luo J, Xu J, Isaacs WB, Bova GS, Yegnasubramanian S. DNA methylation alterations exhibit intraindividual stability and interindividual heterogeneity in prostate cancer metastases. Sci Transl Med. 2013;5(169):169ra10. PMCID: PMC3577373. American Association for the Advancement of Science.
53. Yegnasubramanian S, Haffner MC, Zhang Y, Gurel B, Cornish TC, Wu Z, Irizarry RA, Morgan J, Hicks J, DeWeese TL, Isaacs WB, Bova GS, De Marzo AM, Nelson WG. DNA hypomethylation arises later in prostate cancer progression than CpG island hypermethylation and contributes to metastatic tumor heterogeneity. Cancer Res. 2008;68(21):8954–67. PMCID: PMC2577392.
54. Campagna D, Cope L, Lakkur SS, Henderson C, Laheru D, Iacobuzio-Donahue CA. Gene expression profiles associated with advanced pancreatic cancer. Int J Clin Exp Pathol. 2008;1(1):32–43. PMCID: PMC2480531. e-Century Publishing Corporation.
55. Kim M-S, Pinto SM, Getnet D, Nirujogi RS, Manda SS, Chaerkady R, Madugundu AK, Kelkar DS, Isserlin R, Jain S, Thomas JK, Muthusamy B, Leal-Rojas P, Kumar P, Sahasrabuddhe NA, Balakrishnan L, Advani J, George B, Renuse S, Selvan LDN, Patil AH, Nanjappa V, Radhakrishnan A, Prasad S, Subbannayya T, Raju R, Kumar M, Sreenivasamurthy SK, Marimuthu A, Sathe GJ, Chavan S, Datta KK, Subbannayya Y, Sahu A, Yelamanchi SD, Jayaram S, Rajagopalan P, Sharma J, Murthy KR, Syed N, Goel R, Khan AA, Ahmad S, Dey G, Mudgal K, Chatterjee A, Huang T-C, Zhong J, Wu X, Shaw PG, et al. A draft map of the human proteome. Nature. 2014;509(7502):575–81. PMCID: PMC4403737. Nature Publishing Group.
56. Yachida S, Zhong Y, Patrascu R, Davis MB, Morsberger LA, Griffin CA, Hruban RH, Laheru D, Iacobuzio-Donahue CA. Establishment and characterization of a new cell line, A99, from a primary small cell carcinoma of the pancreas. Pancreas. 2011;40(6):905–10. PMCID: PMC3180880.
57. Monje M, Mitra SS, Freret ME, Raveh TB, Kim J, Masek M, Attema JL, Li G, Haddix T, Edwards MSB, Fisher PG, Weissman IL, Rowitch DH, Vogel H, Wong AJ, Beachy PA. Hedgehog-responsive candidate cell of origin for diffuse intrinsic pontine glioma. Proc Natl Acad Sci U S A. 2011;108(11):4453–8. PMCID: PMC3060250. National Academy of Sciences.
58. Caretti V, Sewing ACP, Lagerweij T, Schellen P, Bugiani M, Jansen MHA, van Vuurden DG, Navis AC, Horsman I, Vandertop WP, Noske DP, Wesseling P, Kaspers GJL, Nazarian J, Vogel H, Hulleman E, Monje M, Wurdinger T. Human pontine glioma cells can induce murine tumors. Acta Neuropathol. 2014;127(6):897–909. PMCID: PMC4135053. Springer Berlin Heidelberg.

59. Hooper JE, Cantor EL, Ehlen MS, Banerjee A, Malempati S, Stenzel P, Woltjer RL, Gandour-Edwards R, Goodwin NC, Yang Y, Kaur P, Bult CJ, Airhart SD, Keller C. A patient-derived xenograft model of parameningeal embryonal rhabdomyosarcoma for preclinical studies. Sarcoma. 2015;2015(3):826124–7. PMCID: PMC4677247. Hindawi.
60. Arnold MA, Barr FG. Molecular diagnostics in the management of rhabdomyosarcoma. Expert Rev Mol Diagn. 2017;17(2):189–94. PMCID: PMC5657295.
61. Start RD, McCulloch TA, Benbow EW, Lauder I, Underwood JC. Clinical necropsy rates during the 1980s: the continued decline. J Pathol. 1993;171(1):63–6. Wiley-Blackwell.
62. Bova GS, Kallio HML, Annala M, Kivinummi K, Högnäs G, Häyrynen S, Rantapero T, Kivinen V, Isaacs WB, Tolonen T, Nykter M, Visakorpi T. Integrated clinical, whole-genome, and transcriptome analysis of multisampled lethal metastatic prostate cancer. Cold Spring Harb Mol Case Stud. 2016;2(3):a000752. PMCID: PMC4853517. Cold Spring Harbor Laboratory Press.
63. Ritchie MD, Holzinger ER, Li R, Pendergrass SA, Kim D. Methods of integrating data to uncover genotype-phenotype interactions. Nat Rev Genet. 2015;16(2):85–97. Nature Publishing Group.

9 Performance of Rapid Research Autopsy

Jody E. Hooper and Eleonora Duregon

Introduction

As outlined in the previous chapter, the concept of utilizing autopsy as a unique opportunity for tissue sampling is spreading across the United States and internationally. Rapid autopsies (sometimes referred to as postmortem tissue donation or, less attractively, as "warm" autopsies) can provide tissue specimens in large volumes and can sample across numerous anatomic locations simultaneously, including inaccessible sites such as bony metastases, brain, or spinal cord lesions [1]. With post diagnostic biopsy or resection often being impossible in patients with widely disseminated disease, autopsy is the best key to the study of tumor and disease heterogeneity. Institutional rapid autopsy programs for body as well as brain sampling have been well described in the past two decades [1–11] and have previously led to significant advances in cancer research in the areas of prostate [1, 2, 4–6, 11], pancreas [9], breast [7], and pediatric brain tumors [3, 8, 10]. This chapter will review practical considerations in development, growth, and maintenance of a rapid autopsy program. Best practices for collaboration with researchers, composition of rapid autopsy teams, autopsy logistics and procedures, and sample collection techniques will be explained.

J. E. Hooper (✉) · E. Duregon
Department of Pathology, The Johns Hopkins University, Baltimore, MD, USA
e-mail: jhooper9@jhmi.edu; eduregо1@jhmi.edu

J. E. Hooper, A. K. Williamson (eds.), *Autopsy in the 21st Century*,
https://doi.org/10.1007/978-3-319-98373-8_9

Current Rapid Autopsy Programs

Rapid autopsy programs (RAP) began in the late 1980s by focusing on brain biobanking. Current programs for body postmortem sampling are mainly, though not exclusively, located at university centers. There are programs in various regions of North America (Table 9.1), Canada, and Australia, with recently developing programs in the United Kingdom and Germany. Most centers concentrate on cancer, usually focusing on only one or two organ systems, but there are several centralized and generalized programs interacting with researchers in all organ systems, including at Johns Hopkins University and Memorial Sloan Kettering Cancer Center. However, some programs also focus on other types of disease such as pulmonary idiopathic fibrosis, Alzheimer disease, multiple sclerosis, or scleroderma [12, 13]. Any systemic disease where research could benefit from the power to sample multiple or inaccessible sites can be studied using rapid autopsy samples.

A RAP is a complex and labor-intensive organism. Although each center has its own particularities depending on its location, state laws, organization, and

Table 9.1 Overview of rapid autopsy programs in North America

Institution	Location (City/state)	Year program Began	Tissue collected
Banner Health	Phoenix, AZ	1987	1987–2005 brain only 2005 all tumor types
University Health Network	Toronto, Canada	2012/2013	All tumor types
Johns Hopkins University	Baltimore, MD	2000	2000 prostate, pancreas, and breast 2014 all tumor types
Massachusetts General	Boston, MA	2016	All tumor types
Memorial Sloan Kettering	New York, NY	2015	All tumor types
University of Michigan	Ann Arbor, MI	1996	All tumor type
University of Nebraska Medical Center	Omaha, NE	2002	Pancreas
NIH/NCI	Bethesda, MD	2013	SCLC, ESCC, pNET, thymic, mesothelioma
University of North Carolina	Chapel Hill, NC	2002	Breast
Ohio State University	Columbus, OH	2013	All tumor types
University of Pittsburgh	Pittsburgh, PA	2003	Lung, heart, vertebral shavings
University of Washington	Seattle, WA	1989	Prostate
University of Washington	Seattle, WA	2008/2009	Brain (reported with prostate, other neuro programs not listed)
Weill Cornell	New York, NY	2013	Metastatic/prostate, cervix, colon, bladder, brain

availability of team members, the duties, infrastructure, and logistics that are necessary for development of a RAP are shared among all centers.

Key Factors for a Rapid Autopsy Program

Delineating Scope of Program and Establishing Researcher Relationships

It is important to clearly define what samples will be taken, how they will be processed, and who will participate at the time of the autopsy and after it, particularly in programs where the sampling pathologist or technician is not also the researcher. *Unlike other venues, in rapid autopsy the limiting factor is not the amount of tissue available but the time and resources available for collection.*

Successful collaboration between clinicians and researchers can be broken down into a series of action steps (Fig. 9.1). The concept of utilizing postmortem tissue and the potentially available quantities of tissue is new enough to some researchers that careful a priori thought is required about how the RAP could fit into existing projects or create new avenues for investigation (CONSIDER). The patient population and sample type must be determined. As detailed in Chap. 8, postmortem intervals can markedly affect how tissue may be utilized, and parameters for different case scenarios should be delineated (DEFINE, MEET). The rapid autopsy program must be

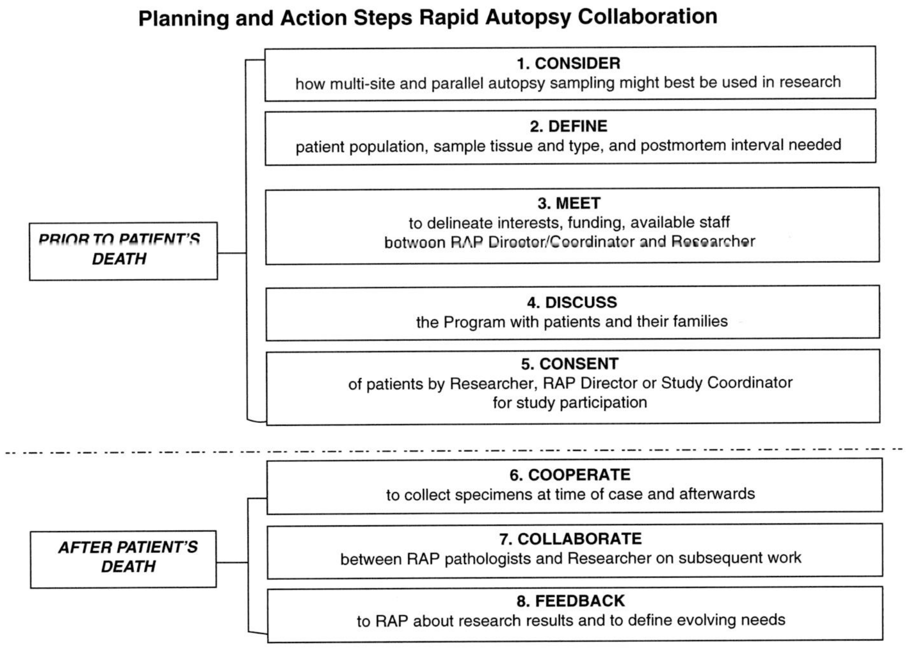

Fig. 9.1 Planning and action steps for successful rapid autopsy collaboration

reviewed with potential participants and families (DISCUSS) and proper legal documents acquired (CONSENT). Researchers and pathologists or other scientists who perform the rapid autopsy must work together (COOPERATE) prior to and at the time of collection and during evaluation and subsequent research (COLLABORATE). Lastly, rapid autopsy pathologists should create a communication loop about research results, family experiences, and evolving case needs (FEEDBACK).

Identifying Participants in the Program: How and When

Patients who decide to participate in a RAP may be referred by clinicians or hospice workers, may have existing relationships with researchers in the field of their cancer or disease, or may seek out programs on the internet themselves. It is important for RAP program directors to have active relationships with treating clinicians in the disease of interest. It is often valuable for the pathologist to speak to tumor boards, research collaboration groups, and in Grand Rounds venues to introduce the idea of postmortem tissue collection and the specifics of the available program. Outreach for programs can include participation in cancer-focused events, websites, and hard copy materials such as brochures which may be distributed in clinic settings.

Although timing of discussion with patients and families must be very individualized, there are two main times when the subject of postmortem donation may be successfully broached. One is at the point when hospice care is being discussed, and the patients and families may be receptive to considering end of life care in general. However, another productive time is much earlier, in the context of research and participation in clinical trials. Rapid autopsy can be offered routinely as another option in the spectrum of possible research involvement. Fruitful relationships can also be built with hospice providers including nurses, social workers, and clergy. These groups often have frequent personal interactions with both patients and their families and can gauge when delicate subjects may be discussed and how to broach the idea of RAP participation in a supportive and sensitive way [14]. It is valuable for a provider known to the patient as well as an autopsy team member who is knowledgeable about the procedure to both be available for questions. The authors have frequently met with patients and families in person at clinic visits or as hospital inpatients after an introduction by a familiar caregiver. These discussions often lead to truly informed consent for the RAP and facilitate arrangement of complex logistics with family members, an important consideration.

Rules Governing Autopsy and Use of Postmortem Tissue

Federal and State Regulations

In the United States, as in much of the world, all medical research on human subjects is ethically and legally guided by the Declaration of Helsinki. Other documents of historical importance include the Nuremberg Code and Declaration of

Geneva. The principles of the Declaration of Helsinki are recognized in the US legal system within the Code of Federal Regulations (CFR) [15] where they are summarized as the Common Rule. The Common Rule is administered by the US Office of Human Research Protection, which exists to ensure that all human subject research will adhere to all appropriate standards. The health information of human subjects is also protected by the Health Insurance Portability and Accountability Act of 1996 (HIPAA), and this protection continues after death. However, the Common Rule applies only to living human subjects, and therefore the US federal government does not directly regulate research performed on deceased human subjects, but rather places responsibility for such regulation on individual states [16]. Each state has its own unique set of laws applicable to research usage of tissue from deceased subjects, but there is commonality in that 48 states have adopted the most recent form of the Uniform Anatomical Gift Act (UAGA). The original UAGA, enacted in 1968, was focused on increasing the availability of donor organs for transplantation, but the 2006 revision (http://www.uniformlaws.org/ActSummary.aspx?title=Anatomical%20Gift%20Act%20(2006)) expressly states that tissue donation may be made for the purposes of transplantation, therapy, research, or education [13]. In most states, the research informed consent (i.e., the Study Consent) for autopsy tissue donation must be obtained prior to the subject's death. Consenting prospective subjects themselves for participation in postmortem research recognizes and advances their premortem choices and maximizes the principle of respect for persons [17]. Therefore, although general research advance directives are at times acceptable, it is highly recommended that established research protocols strive for protocol-specific advance consent from prospective research subjects. When first-person consent is not possible, valid consent from a legally recognized surrogate is sufficient to protect the interests of the deceased. In the United States, the UAGA lists next of kin as the appropriate surrogate for anatomical gifts in the following order of priority: spouse, adult son or daughter, either parent, adult brother or sister, grandparent, or a guardian of the person of the decedent at the time of death. Specific state laws should be consulted to determine whether there is a legally authorized surrogate for decisions about research with the deceased and who that person may be. When legally authorized surrogates disagree, an ethics committee may help resolve the dispute. The multidisciplinary expert Consensus Panel on Research with the Recently Dead (CPRRD) [17] discourages proceeding with research with the dead in cases of disagreement. Moreover, if the authorized surrogate withdraws consent during the course of the research, no further research should be performed or information collected [17].

Difficulties can arise when family members wish to veto an individual's authorization to use his or her own body for research after death. In the United States, the UAGA forbids family veto of the wishes of the person who has authorized the donation of his or her organs while still living, and many state laws now honor donor or "first-person" consent, regardless of the wishes of next of kin. The conventional practice of deferring decisions to family members is based primarily on respect for their feelings in a time of grief [18]. As the family members must live with the consequences and must handle matters that arise after their relative's death, it is crucial to address their concerns, particularly because research with the recently deceased is less widely known and accepted than organ transplantation is. The CPRRD therefore recommends that investigators address the concerns of the family to the satisfaction of the family whenever possible before proceeding.

The Study Consent

The Study Consent should include explicit permission for (1) genetic sequencing, (2) generation of cell lines, (3) tissue banking, (4) sharing of tissue with researchers at other institutions in addition to the host institution, (5) taking images of cases, (6) retrieval of slides and blocks from prior biopsy and resection specimens, and (7) collection of premortem blood specimens, if applicable. It is extremely important that this individualized consent is obtained for postmortem specimens and that it is written in general enough terms to be used for patients with all types of diseases. It appears likely that individualized consent will soon be required for genetic testing and establishing cell lines, even in deceased patients, as regulatory agencies become aware of the expanding potential of postmortem tissue.

In addition to the necessary Study Consent, rapid autopsies require a consent for the autopsy procedure itself, in the same way as regular diagnostic autopsies do. Depending on state law, the autopsy consent can be either signed by the patient himself in advance (this is also the case in the Australian CASCADE Program [19]) or must be signed by the legal next of kin only after the patient dies (this is true for a number of RAPs across the United States including at the Johns Hopkins University, Baltimore, MD, at the University of Michigan, Ann Arbor, MI [2, 20] and at Weill Cornell Medicine, New York, NY [21, 22]). The patient or legal next of kin can specify that the procedure is to be a complete autopsy or restrict the procedure.

Institutional Review Board Permissions and Ethical Considerations

Depending on the state in which the RAP is operating, jurisdictions differ on whether a proposal for research with the newly deceased must be reviewed. In the United States, federal regulations define human subjects as living human beings [23]; thus, the requirement that all human research undergo review by an Institutional Review Board (IRB) does not extend to research with the deceased. This is not the case in other jurisdictions such as Canada, where research with human remains including cadavers requires review and approval by research ethics boards [17]. Regardless of regulatory requirements, the CPRRD recommends review by a multidisciplinary panel in order to address any distinct ethical issues involved in this research. Research with the deceased should proceed only after approval by a properly constituted institutional review board. As a matter of fact, the majority of existing RAPs operate under IRB-reviewed protocols [1, 12, 19, 22, 24].

As has been painfully clear since the Alder Hey affair where organs were retained without the knowledge or permission of the decedent's family [25–27], the research activities that will be performed on tissues collected during a rapid autopsy must be disclosed on both the study and autopsy consents. The CPRRD offers guidelines as direction for conducting ethical research with whole deceased bodies [17] and can be helpful in the development of specific guidelines tailored to an institution's own RAP.

Complete Autopsies Versus Restricted Procedures Versus Tissue Procurement Only

The overt purpose of a RAP is to provide pathologically characterized control and diseased tissue to research scientists, enabling them to discover the underlying genetic and proteomic changes specific to each disease and to design appropriate therapeutic interventions [13]. However, the autopsy examination itself can also discover diagnostic information which can be helpful to families and provide for accurate clinicopathologic correlation. Some RAPs provide a tissue procurement service only, limiting dissection to the researcher's specific needs. This approach is touted by some as saving time or allowing the tissue sampling to be performed by a technician or physician assistant without pathologist involvement. More commonly, in parallel or following the tissue procurement, the autopsy proceeds in accordance with the protocol established by the local autopsy service [1, 21]. An autopsy pathologist can not only synthesize diagnostic information but also can lend sophisticated gross evaluation to the selection of research tissue samples, pinpointing viable areas of malignancy or disease involvement. Conducting a full dissection also allows for the discovery and sampling of previously unknown metastatic sites revealed by the autopsy itself.

The final decision of how complete an autopsy procedure will be resides with the signer of the autopsy consent, though patients and families often will follow guidelines suggested to them by the clinician or researcher. Most cases at the Johns Hopkins RAP are consented as complete autopsies including all organs, brain, eyes, and spinal cord, with special permission for any dissection involving the limbs or face. After research sampling, the autopsy is performed as a regular case would be, with resident participation and preparation of a full diagnostic report. However, it is always important to fully document invasive dissection procedures even when only tissue sampling is performed. This approach allows the families to receive a complete and explanatory report and gives trainees the opportunity to observe disease that they would not normally see, as patients with metastatic cancer often do not die as hospital inpatients.

Logistics for Notification of the Death and Transport of the Patient

In some centers the postmortem interval (PMI) goal for in-house patients is about 1 h [22], while for patients who die at home or hospice, the PMI mainly depends on the distance and consequently the duration of transportation to the hospital. Often patients do die in an inpatient hospice or at home with or without assisting hospice care. While postmortem intervals for standard autopsies are routinely over 24 h and often longer, every effort must be made in a RAP to manage the considerable logistical challenge of transporting the body in a more timely fashion. Many RAPs use a pager system or a dedicated answering service; the latter enables families to use a single 1–800 number to easily reach any of a list of sequential contacts among the RAP team members, ensuring a prompt response when the patient has died. Some programs successfully use a contracted independent funeral home or transport service that is always on call to deliver the patient's body to the autopsy institution. In other cases, advance transportation and logistical planning are individually arranged with out-of-state funeral homes local to home hospice patients. Programs have different standards for what distances from the hospital they will accept and if postmortem autopsy consenting is required, additional time for this must be allotted.

Because prearranged logistics ensure an optimal postmortem interval within the restrictions created by family needs, it is best to identify patients before the immediate preterminal period. This means that there will often be a period of time during which patients will be consented for the study but not in extremis. A rapid autopsy coordinator must walk a fine line between keeping informed about the status of prospective and consented participants and unduly intruding upon patients and families [28]. Hospice workers can often assist with this process.

Best Practices During and After a Rapid Autopsy

Composition of Rapid Autopsy Teams

The multifaceted organization, cost, and labor of a RAP require significant institutional commitment for success. One of the major factors contributing to timely specimen procurement is the availability and composition of the on-call team. A crucial issue to the long-term survival and success of a RAP is to avoid the drain on personnel required to operate the program 15–24 h a day, 365 days a year [29]. Many RAPs fail because, though they initially achieve consistently short PMI, they are understaffed, and this leads to burnout of the team and breakdown of the group [13]. Consequently, RAP logistics need to be flexible and increase the number of personnel to allow for rotational periods on call as the program grows. Programs with many personnel, for example, RAPs operated by oncology researchers who employ numerous laboratory technicians, may choose to frequently rotate coverage on a 24/7 basis, while other programs may choose the approach of using a reduced number of staff available for fewer daily hours.

RAP Examples

Here follow a few examples of well-established RAPs in the United States, their logistics and approaches to staffing. With an average of 90 cases each year, the Sun Health Research Institute [13] in Phoenix, Arizona, limits on-call periods for any one individual to no more than 4 months per year. They use four rotating on-call teams, each team consisting of two trained dissectors (one each for the brain and body, working in parallel) and two assistants. The trained dissectors are employees of the institute, while the assistants are derived from volunteers among the entire scientific institute and technical and administrative staff. Generally, all procedures are completed in 3–4 h, and the total time a team member typically spends on a call, including transportation to and from his or her home, is between 3 and 5 h.

At the University of Nebraska Medical Center, a rotating research team is available 24 h, 7 days a week consisting of two full-time technicians, with participation of three on-call technicians and pathology assistants [29]. The RAP of the University of Michigan at Ann Arbor, Michigan, consists of two teams, an autopsy team and a tissue procurement team, which are alerted and work together during each case, and all are available 24/7. The autopsy team consists of a staff genitourinary pathologist, genitourinary pathology fellow, pathology resident, and a pathology assistant. The tissue procurement team consists of the medical oncologist, staff and postdoctoral researchers, laboratory assistants, and a urology resident [1]. At Weill Cornell, the RAP team comprises an attending autopsy pathologist, a pathology resident, an autopsy technical assistant, and 2–4 additional members including pathologists, postdoctoral researchers, and research technicians who aid in tissue procurement and initial processing. The team may also include the patient's treating oncologists and surgeons [22]. The Johns Hopkins RAP team in Baltimore, Maryland, consists of a pathologist/RAP director, a specimen coordinator, an autopsy assistant/diener to assist in dissection, and a pathologist research autopsy fellow, as well as various subspecialty research team members. During daytime hours, a physician's assistant, pathology photography representative, and a resident on regular rotation will participate. The core team is available 7 days a week for 15 h per day.

Available space and physical resources will contribute to short postmortem intervals and case times. The Johns Hopkins RAP team pre-creates a templated sheet for each patient at the time of study consenting that includes demographic information and medical history including last imaging and all lesions planned to be targeted. Where possible, pre-labeling of containers and bags is also highly helpful if there is sufficient space for storage [13]. Direct affiliation with an autopsy service is helpful as equipment and refrigeration may be required.

Sample Prioritization and Selection

Each rapid autopsy is a powerful opportunity to supply multiple researchers with many valuable specimens at the same time. As an example, at the Johns Hopkins RAP, a single rapid autopsy case can provide tumor tissue to Johns Hopkins researchers, tissue to three other out-of-state institutions (including NIH), and banked tissue for the program itself, as well as normal controls of the brain, eye, pituitary, heart, pancreatic duct, and skeletal muscle for other research groups. To accomplish this type of multifaceted action during a case, it is imperative to have prearranged sampling protocols which specify types of tissue and processing methods. At Hopkins, each research group has a designated representative, and these people are contacted as a group as soon as the patient's death is reported. Research teams provide supplemental personnel, with the extent and composition of these teams varying by the number of specimens sought and the extent of immediate on-site processing required. It can also be highly useful to sample each lesion or normal tissue in parallel by allocating part of the same area to be collected fresh in media such as RPMI, part flash frozen in liquid nitrogen or gradually frozen in OCT, and part fixed in formalin. Corresponding studies utilizing cell lines or xenografts, sequencing, and immunohistochemical staining can create synergy, helping to delineate the "life cycle" of a cancer cell. It is important to have at least one team member exclusively dedicated to specimen labeling and tracking to facilitate this important parallel sampling.

Post-case activities usually include the review of all histologic sections of metastatic samples and normal control tissues and recording the percentage of neoplastic tissue, viable tumor, and other cells. For specific cases, PowerPoint slides are prepared that summarize the clinical history of the patient, the rapid autopsy findings with photomicrographs, the analysis of tissue viability, and the timing of tissue sampling. This material can then be circulated among the members of both the autopsy and research teams. One month after the autopsy, a joint meeting is held by the two teams to review rapid autopsy findings, make clinicopathologic correlations, and discuss planning for follow-up genetic and other studies utilizing the samples.

Tissue Sampling Processes

Experience has shown that contamination by bacteria and fungi can be significant obstacles to establishment of cell lines and xenografts in postmortem sampling, in particular because the autopsy suite is not a sterile environment even after standard disinfection [30]. Of twenty-four rapid autopsies performed by the first author at a previous institution, the first seven cases proved to have contaminated samples, mostly by fungal forms. Post collection antibiotics/antifungals in media are helpful; however, proper sterile technique at the time of the autopsy has been the single most important factor in avoiding contamination in the experience of many centers. For this reason, the skin should be either cleaned along the lines of incision with povidone-iodine swabs or the body may be sprayed with ethanol. The best practice calls for full-sized instruments for evisceration, sterilized in a tabletop sterilizer such as is typically used in a dentist's office. In addition, rib cutters rather than a rotating saw are strongly recommended for removing the chest plate, to avoid contamination of the cavity by bone dust. Blood may be obtained through the femoral vessels or by opening the pericardium, cleaning the surface of the heart and great vessels with alcohol, and puncturing the inferior vena cava and ventricles with a 16-gauge needle and syringe.

The sampling process is generally performed by one or more pathologists or assistants using disposable sterile blades and forceps (one set per tumor site) with care to avoid areas of grossly evident necrosis or hemorrhage and can follow one of two methods. In the first approach, organs are removed from the body en bloc, weighed, reviewed systematically for macroscopic evidence of disease, and then sectioned. The normal tissues and metastatic sites are then dissected and sampled. Care in selection of lesions is important in that frequently smaller metastases (2–4 cm) show better viability than larger tumors that often have central necrosis. Certain centers spray samples with ethanol before putting them in media [19]. In the second approach, as many lesions as possible are sampled in situ using disposable sterile instruments after opening of the chest and abdomen with minimal manipulation of the bowel. Samples are placed on a cart covered by a sterile drape, which is used as a clean working surface for immediate further dissection. The organ block may then be removed and further dissection carried out to obtain additional lesions that may be difficult to reach from an anterior approach, such as adrenal gland metastases. In a protocol first developed at the University of Washington, a hollow point drill with a sterilizable orthopedic bit may be used to obtain cores from the axial and appendicular skeleton without disturbing the overall frame of the body [1]. Date of collection, time of processing, and the location of all biological samples should be recorded on a standard form.

Timing and Processing of Samples

Since their beginning, the overriding organizing principle for all RAPs has been that the samples or organs must be removed and processed as rapidly as possible. With this press for "high-quality" tissue comes the need to determine the critical markers of quality for human postmortem tissue [31]. The postmortem interval (PMI) is defined as the time elapsing between the time of death and the time the tissue has been placed in the preservative (either medium for fresh samples, snap freezing in liquid nitrogen, or fixation in formalin). Depending on the center and the particular aspects of the case involved, PMI can range between 0.5 and 23 h. Postmortem tissue quality is affected by PMI, premortem (agonal) conditions, and other postmortem factors. Traditionally, a low PMI has been the hallmark of high tissue quality [32–36].

Though the effect of PMI on sampling outcomes can be highly individualized by the type of cancer or disease and patient body habitus, some general PMI guidelines for successful sampling can be gleaned from the literature (see also Chap. 8). As depicted in Fig. 9.2, fresh samples with living cells are best gathered within 6–8 h of death. Specimens for RNA and DNA sequencing may be frozen or placed in a media with stabilizing reagent and are generally best collected within 12 h of death at most. Histology and immunohistochemistry will still produce good results after 12 h of PMI. The author has had the experience of cell lines growing from a sample taken after 12 h when the setting (within an area of hemorrhage) was propitious. Rapid autopsy programs and researchers should discuss together what collections will be done if circumstances (family concerns, weather, or traffic) extend the postmortem interval longer than planned.

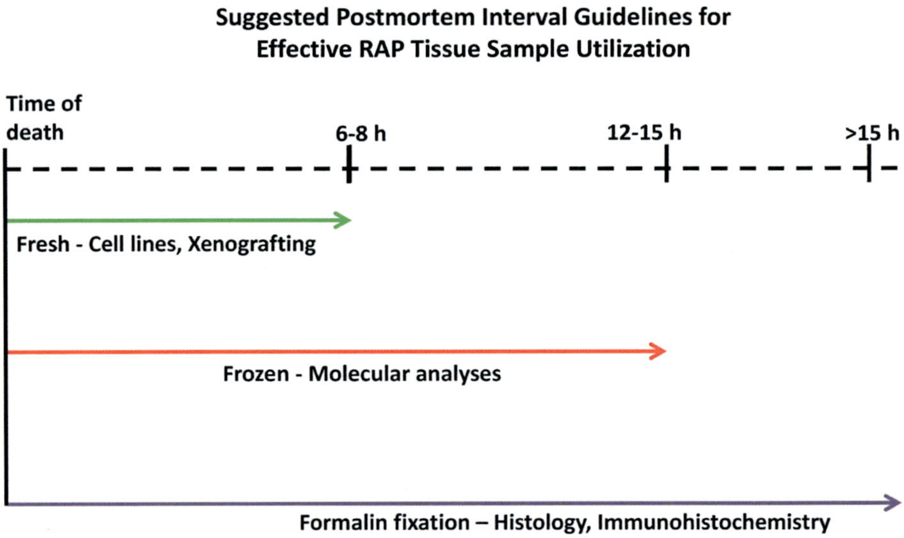

Fig. 9.2 Suggested postmortem interval guidelines for effective RAP tissue sample utilization

Specimens for cell cultures and xenografting should be harvested in sterilely tittered Roswell Park Memorial Institute (RPMI) medium, which may have added antibiotics or antifungals. Some protocols for fresh tissue harvesting require the tumor tissue be washed in a solution of HBSS or with 5.0% antibiotic/antimycotic additive [1] or washed in hydrogen peroxide and PBS before being placed in the medium. Once in appropriate medium and kept at refrigerated temperatures (35 °F/1.6 °C), specimens may be shipped without compromising the development of cell lines or patient-derived xenografts. Fresh tissue specimens may also be frozen in optimal cutting temperature (OCT) compound with cryomolds or in dry ice for later thawing, after which recovered cells are typically still intact.

Normal and malignant tissues are usually collected as frozen tissue for future molecular studies such as RNA/DNA sequencing or proteomic or metabolomics studies. Specimens can either be placed in OCT media or snap frozen in liquid nitrogen in 1.5 ml cryovials or 50 mL tubes, which in both cases are then stored at −80 °C. Specimens corresponding to those collected in liquid nitrogen are also fixed in 10% buffered formalin and paraffin embedded. Histologic sections stained with hematoxylin and eosin can then be prepared and evaluated, especially to verify the amount of viable neoplastic tissue present in each sample. Usually paraffin blocks are stored at room temperature in archival files. It is well documented that storing slides at room temperature is detrimental for antibody immunoreactivity for several antigens [37–40] compared with leaving the tissue in the paraffin blocks and storing them at room temperature. However, studies have shown decreased staining of at least some immunohistochemistry-based markers related to increased paraffin block age, as well [41, 42]. Marked reduction in RNA in situ signaling has been documented after storage of blocks for 5 years and even in some cases after 1 year [40].

Several techniques have been suggested to preserve reactivity in unstained slides. One option is to coat slides with paraffin to simulate leaving slides in the protective confines of the paraffin block [38, 43], though with this approach there is still a slight decrease in immunoreactivity with paraffin removal. Another suggested technique is to freeze unstained slides at −20 °C, which has been shown to preserve in situ hybridization even more effectively than storage within the block [40, 44]. Since additional studies are needed to address whether storing unstained slides or paraffin blocks at −20 °C can preserve protein immunogenicity most effectively, the numerous specimens collected in parallel as part of a rapid autopsy protocol offer great opportunities for further research and evaluation.

Rapid Autopsy Case Illustration

Following is a complete description of a rapid autopsy case at the authors' institution, detailing the processes and events before, during, and after the rapid autopsy. Certain details of the case have been changed to protect patient privacy and enhance the instructional value provided.

Background

The patient was a 57-year-old man with widely metastatic BRAF wild-type melanoma with the *cKit* L576 mutation. The melanoma was initially diagnosed 4 years prior to autopsy as an ulcerated lesion on the right cheek which was excised with a negative sentinel node biopsy. He completed chemotherapy but developed multiple metastases 2 years later. He was study consented by the rapid autopsy program director during an outpatient clinic visit after an introduction by his treating clinician. Three months after consenting, he died at his home and was pronounced at 4:00 AM of that day. His legal next of kin signed and faxed the autopsy consent to the director of the rapid autopsy program by 5:30 AM of that same day. The patient arrived in the autopsy suite at 8:45 AM, and the autopsy began at 9:00 AM, 5 h after death. The rapid autopsy was attended by the RAP director (lead pathologist), an autopsy assistant (diener), a specimen coordinator, one pathology postdoctoral fellow, two research associates of the melanoma oncology team, and a dedicated pathology photographer. The photographer was available because the case took place during daytime hours; otherwise photographs would have been taken by the specimen coordinator.

Examination Findings

The external examination was that of a cachectic Caucasian man. After disinfection of the skin surface with povidone-iodine swabs, a standard Y-shaped incision was made with a sterile scalpel from the anterior axillary line to the sternum and down to the pubic bone. A 10 × 10 × 5 cm dark brown friable mass was found on the anterior right chest wall extending to the right axilla, eroding through ribs and into the right upper lobe of the lung (Fig. 9.3a, b). There was an associated 6 × 5 cm area of small brown nodules studding the pleural surface of the chest wall with parasternal lymphadenopathy. The left lung had a 3 cm dark brown nodule adjacent to the left upper lobe and adherent to the pulmonary vein, without gross invasion into the vein. The omentum was caked and adherent to the small intestine and had an 8 cm solid and cystic dark brown mass abutting the greater curvature of the stomach. In the left lower quadrant of the abdomen, within the area of omental caking, a 6.5 × 4 cm solid dark brown mass was adherent to the pelvic side wall, the serosa of colon, and eroding through the small intestine. Further numerous dark brown nodules were present in the omentum, mesentery, and abdominal wall (Fig. 9.3c).

Sampling Procedure

The lead pathologist sampled all readily accessible metastatic sites with sterile scalpel and forceps, using fresh instruments for each site. Normal tissue controls were sampled in situ by the same method. Samples were placed on the dedicated cart covered by a sterile surgical drape and dissected by the postdoctoral fellow. She guided the tissue sampling, avoiding macroscopically evident necrotic areas, and

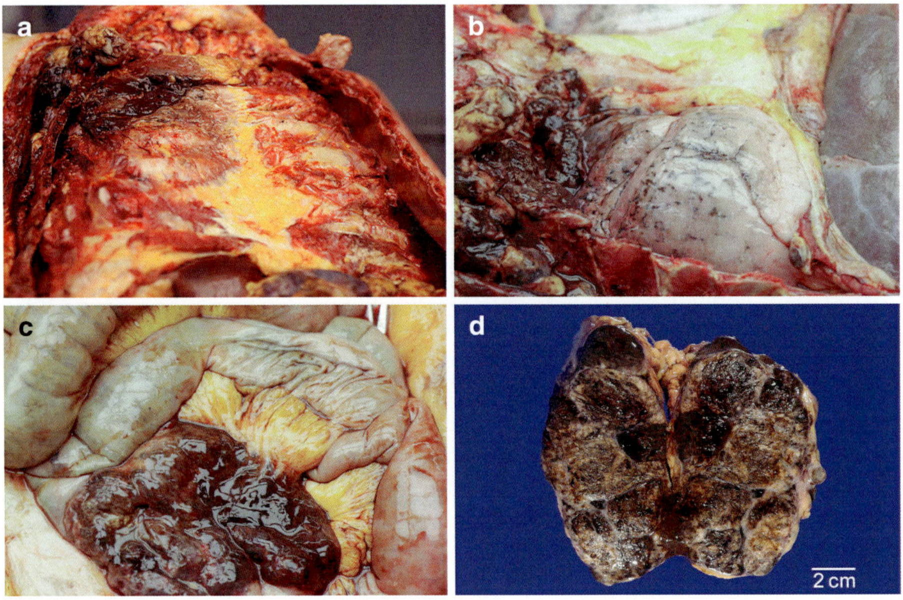

Fig. 9.3 Gross images from rapid autopsy case example. (**a**) Pigmented right chest wall mass eroding ribs and spreading to axilla, (**b**) right upper lobe lung mass, (**c**) pigmented mass in mesentery of small intestine, (**d**) right adrenal gland entirely replaced by an approximately 9 cm pigmented mass

then distributed minced metastatic tissues to the melanoma oncology team research associates. Fresh samples for cell culture were taken first with corresponding specimens snap frozen in liquid nitrogen and fixed in 10% neutral buffered formalin for routine histologic processing. The specimen coordinator recorded all sample locations and dates and times of collection on specimen tubes and a specimen manifest. After full in situ sampling including normal tissue controls, all of the organs were removed from the body en bloc, weighed, and sectioned at every 1–2 cm. The right lung showed an extension of the dark brown chest mass into the upper lobe. The stomach contained multiple dark brown nodules, merging to confluence in some areas and ranging in size from 2 to 5 cm. The mucosa of the small intestine contained five scattered variegated tan brown nodules ranging in size from 1.0 to 4.5 cm. The liver contained multiple variegated to dark brown nodules up to 3 cm in size, the largest in the lateral right lobe. In the peripancreatic soft tissues, a 5.2 × 1.5 cm mass of lymph nodes was found. The left ureter was encased in a circumferential brown mass without obstruction or hydronephrosis. The adrenal glands were bilaterally entirely replaced by numerous variegated pale to dark brown nodules (Fig. 9.3d). The thyroid gland had a 2 cm dark brown nodule in the left inferior pole. All of the other organs, including the brain and spinal cord, were unremarkable.

Summary of Case

The first research specimens were collected at 9:30 AM and the last at 10:25 AM. Fresh samples were taken from ten malignant sites including the right chest wall, various liver metastases, right axillary lymph node, lungs, pancreas, stomach, and abdomen. Ten metastatic sites (liver, peripancreatic soft tissue, lower abdominal mass, right and left lung, right and left adrenal gland, small intestine, thyroid, stomach) and 11 normal tissues (skin, skeletal muscle, fat, heart, left lung, pancreas, kidney, liver, spleen, thyroid, and adrenal gland) were sampled, all having tissue frozen as well as fixed in formalin for paraffin embedding. Fresh samples were also shipped to a separate research group outside of the institution on the same afternoon.

Post-Case Activities

The postdoctoral fellow reviewed all histologic sections of metastatic samples and normal control tissues, recording the percentage of melanoma, viable melanoma, and viable cells for other tissues. Microscopic evidence of melanoma was found in the left and right upper lobes of the lungs, gastric mucosa, liver, peripancreatic soft tissues, omentum, small and large bowel mucosa, left renal ureter, bilateral adrenal glands, and thyroid. The liver metastases were the most necrotic among all of those collected. The lead pathologist prepared PowerPoint slides that summarized the clinical history of the patient, the rapid autopsy findings with photomicrographs, the analysis of tissue viability, and the timing of tissue sampling. This material was then circulated among the members of both the autopsy and melanoma research teams. One month after the autopsy, a joint meeting was held by the two teams to review the rapid autopsy findings, make clinical-pathologic correlations, and discuss planning for follow-up genetic and other studies utilizing the samples. Images of histology and growing cell lines (verified to be positive for melanoma markers by flow cytometry) from the right chest lesion were shared at this meeting (Fig. 9.4).

Value to Patients and Families

Growing numbers of patients with cancer or chronic disease are expressing interest in donating tissues, organs, or their bodies after death, even independently of clinicians or hospice workers' initial introduction of the topic. Some cancer patients see this as an opportunity to fulfill commitments as organ donors, and a majority state it is a way to "give back" to medical research and to the community [45]. In 60

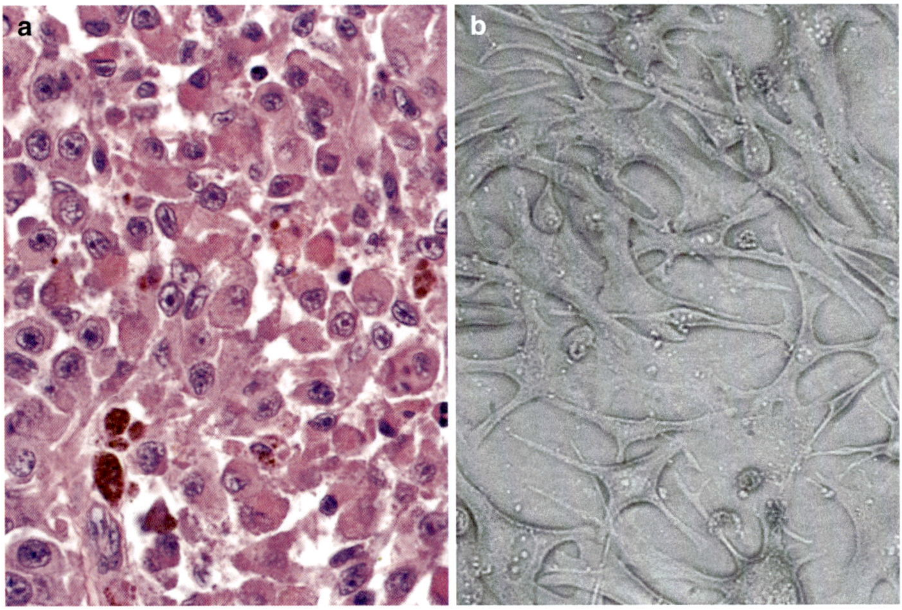

Fig. 9.4 Post rapid autopsy case research images. (**a**) Right chest wall mass, H&E, 400×. Classic morphology of melanoma is observed, with atypical nuclei, large nucleoli, and abundant eosinophilic cytoplasm. Note the good preservation of nuclear membranes and chromatin. (**b**) A right chest wall melanoma metastasis obtained approximately 6 h postmortem was enzymatically digested, and the melanoma cell line "MA2-mel" was established in culture. A photograph was captured after 44 days and two culture passages. After 30 passages in vitro, MA2-mel maintained expression of the melanoma-associated antigens tyrosinase and MART-1 and the cell surface chondroitin sulfate proteoglycan NG2, by 100% of cells as assessed by flow cytometry. Images courtesy of Tracee L. McMiller and Suzanne L. Topalian, Johns Hopkins Bloomberg~Kimmel Institute for Cancer Immunotherapy

interviews surveying the families of children with cancer, 93% of parents either did consent or would have consented to a research autopsy, and none thought that the choice had done harm. They cited learning of medical advances made through research as a positive contribution which would honor the deceased child. Interestingly, over half of those sampled cited apparent physician reluctance to request autopsy as the major barrier to accomplishing postmortem tissue donation [14]. Many parents have also indicated a desire for more specific information about the autopsy procedure [46]. Patients and families possess a tremendous altruistic desire to help others with disease and to advance scientific knowledge [46, 47]. Documentation of the extent of disease can also often help families come to terms with the death and, frequently, the decision to have placed their loved one on comfort measures [48]. It is also important to note that many patients and families desire some form of public recognition for their contribution and most also express interest in receiving follow-up information about the results of research [45]. The authors sponsor a memorial section of the home program website for those families who wish to participate and have links to research results online as well.

Final Thoughts

Creating, developing, and maintaining a full rapid research autopsy program require resources, technical skill at several levels, and motivation, but the opportunities it represents are absolutely unique. It is important to realize that supporting a full-scale program is not the only way to participate in the collection of postmortem research tissue. To provide this valuable service to all researchers, patients, and families who are seeking it will require not only established full service programs at major hospital and university centers but also innovative solutions such as sample retrieval kits which can be sent to smaller centers or even private pathology practices.

Rapid autopsy is a thoroughly modern purpose for an otherwise ancient technique and a chance for the practitioner of autopsy to demonstrate extraordinary value in a fresh way. While a rapid autopsy supplies tissue for developing new genomic and proteomic studies, it can and should also fulfill the worthy purposes that all autopsies can fulfill: those of diagnostic accuracy, education, training, and information and closure for family members.

References

1. Rubin MA, Putzi M, Mucci N, et al. Rapid ("warm") autopsy study for procurement of metastatic prostate cancer. Clin Cancer Res. 2000;6(3):1038–45.
2. Shah RB, Mehra R, Chinnaiyan AM, et al. Androgen-independent prostate cancer is a heterogeneous group of diseases: lessons from a rapid autopsy program. Cancer Res. 2004;64(24):9209–16.
3. Zarghooni M, Bartels U, Lee E, et al. Whole-genome profiling of pediatric diffuse intrinsic pontine gliomas highlights platelet-derived growth factor receptor alpha and poly (ADP-ribose) polymerase as potential therapeutic targets. J Clin Oncol. 2010;28(8):1337–44.

4. Esgueva R, Park K, Kim R, et al. Next-generation prostate cancer biobanking: toward a processing protocol amenable for the international cancer genome consortium. Diagn Mol Pathol. 2012;21(2):61–8.
5. Udager AM, Shi Y, Tomlins SA, et al. Frequent discordance between ERG gene rearrangement and ERG protein expression in a rapid autopsy cohort of patients with lethal, metastatic, castration-resistant prostate cancer. Prostate. 2014;74(12):1199–208.
6. Beltran H, Eng K, Mosquera JM, et al. Whole-exome sequencing of metastatic Cancer and biomarkers of treatment response. JAMA Oncol. 2015;1(4):466–74.
7. Juric D, Castel P, Griffith M, et al. Convergent loss of PTEN leads to clinical resistance to a PI(3)Kα inhibitor. Nature. 2015;518(7538):240–4.
8. Kambhampati M, Perez JP, Yadavilli S, et al. A standardized autopsy procurement allows for the comprehensive study of DIPG biology. Oncotarget. 2015;6(14):12740–7.
9. Xie T, Musteanu M, Lopez-Casas PP, et al. Whole exome sequencing of rapid autopsy tumors and xenograft models reveals possible driver mutations underlying tumor progression. PLoS One. 2015;10(11):e0142631.
10. Hoffman LM, DeWire M, Ryall S, et al. Spatial genomic heterogeneity in diffuse intrinsic pontine and midline high-grade glioma: implications for diagnostic biopsy and targeted therapeutics. Acta Neuropathol Commun. 2016;4:1.
11. Beltran H, Prandi D, Mosquera JM, et al. Divergent clonal evolution of castration-resistant neuroendocrine prostate cancer. Nat Med. 2016;22(3):298–305.
12. Lindell KO, Erlen JA, Kaminski N. Lessons from our patients: development of a warm autopsy program. PLoS Med. 2006;3(7):e234.
13. Beach TG, Adler CH, Sue LI, et al. Arizona study of aging and neurodegenerative disorders and brain and body donation program. Neuropathology. 2015;35(4):354–89.
14. Alabran JL, Hooper JE, Hill M, et al. Overcoming autopsy barriers in pediatric cancer research. Pediatr Blood Cancer. 2013;60(2):204–9.
15. Allen MJ, Powers ML, Gronowski KS, Gronowski AM. Human tissue ownership and use in research: what laboratorians and researchers should know. Clin Chem. 2010;56(11):1675–82.
16. Nelkin D, Andrews L. Do the dead have interests? Policy issues for research after life. Am J Law Med. 1998;24(2–3):261–91.
17. Pentz RD, Cohen CB, Wicclair M, et al. Ethics guidelines for research with the recently dead. Nat Med. 2005;11(11):1145–9.
18. Wendler D, Dickert N. The consent process for cadaveric organ procurement: how does it work? How can it be improved? JAMA. 2001;285(3):329–33.
19. Alsop K, Thorne H, Sandhu S, et al. A community-based model of rapid autopsy in end-stage cancer patients. Nat Biotechnol. 2016;34(10):1010–4.
20. Rubin DT, Huo D, Kinnucan JA, et al. Inflammation is an independent risk factor for colonic neoplasia in patients with ulcerative colitis: a case-control study. Clin Gastroenterol Hepatol. 2013;11(12):1601–8. e1601–1604.
21. Faltas BM, Prandi D, Tagawa ST, et al. Clonal evolution of chemotherapy-resistant urothelial carcinoma. Nat Genet. 2016;48(12):1490–9.
22. Pisapia DJ, Salvatore S, Pauli C, et al. Next-generation rapid autopsies enable tumor evolution tracking and generation of preclinical models. JCO Precis Oncol. 2017; https://doi.org/10.1200/PO.16.00038JCO.
23. Protection of human subjects: subpart A. Federal policy for the protection of human subjects. 45 CFR Part 46.102 (f) and 21 CFR50.3 (g).
24. Broniscer A, Baker JN, Baker SJ, et al. Prospective collection of tissue samples at autopsy in children with diffuse intrinsic pontine glioma. Cancer. 2010;116(19):4632–7.
25. Burton JL, Wells M. The Alder Hey affair: implications for pathology practice. J Clin Pathol. 2001;54(11):820–3.
26. Evans HM. What's wrong with "retained organs"? Some personal reflections in the afterglow of "Alder Hey". J Clin Pathol. 2001;54(11):824–6.
27. van Diest PJ, Lopes Cardoso NW, Niesing J. Cadaveric tissue donation: a pathologist's perspective. J Med Ethics. 2003;29(3):135–6.

28. Savas P, Teo ZL, Lefevre C, et al. The subclonal architecture of metastatic breast cancer: results from a prospective community-based rapid autopsy program "CASCADE". PLoS Med. 2016;13(12):e1002204.
29. Ghorpade A, Bruch L, Persidsky Y, et al. Development of a rapid autopsy program for studies of brain immunity. J Neuroimmunol. 2005;163(1–2):135–44.
30. Hostiuc S, Curca GC, Ceausu M, Rusu MC, Niculescu E, Dermengiu D. Infectious risks in autopsy practice. Rom J Leg Med. 2011;19(3):6.
31. Hargrove JL, Schmidt FH. The role of mRNA and protein stability in gene expression. FASEB J. 1989;3(12):2360–70.
32. Barton AJ, Pearson RC, Najlerahim A, Harrison PJ. Pre- and postmortem influences on brain RNA. J Neurochem. 1993;61(1):1–11.
33. Harrison PJ, Heath PR, Eastwood SL, Burnet PW, McDonald B, Pearson RC. The relative importance of premortem acidosis and postmortem interval for human brain gene expression studies: selective mRNA vulnerability and comparison with their encoded proteins. Neurosci Lett. 1995;200(3):151–4.
34. Lewis DA. The human brain revisited: opportunities and challenges in postmortem studies of psychiatric disorders. Neuropsychopharmacology. 2002;26(2):143–54.
35. Trotter SA, Brill LB, Bennett JP. Stability of gene expression in postmortem brain revealed by cDNA gene array analysis. Brain Res. 2002;942(1–2):120–3.
36. Ferrer-Alcón M, La Harpe R, Guimón J, García-Sevilla JA. Downregulation of neuronal cdk5/p35 in opioid addicts and opiate-treated rats: relation to neurofilament phosphorylation. Neuropsychopharmacology. 2003;28(5):947–55.
37. Jacobs TW, Prioleau JE, Stillman IE, Schnitt SJ. Loss of tumor marker-immunostaining intensity on stored paraffin slides of breast cancer. J Natl Cancer Inst. 1996;88(15):1054–9.
38. DiVito KA, Charette LA, Rimm DL, Camp RL. Long-term preservation of antigenicity on tissue microarrays. Lab Investig. 2004;84(8):1071–8.
39. Fergenbaum JH, Garcia-Closas M, Hewitt SM, Lissowska J, Sakoda LC, Sherman ME. Loss of antigenicity in stored sections of breast cancer tissue microarrays. Cancer Epidemiol Biomark Prev. 2004;13(4):667–72.
40. Baena-Del Valle JA, Zheng Q, Hicks JL, et al. Rapid loss of RNA detection by in situ hybridization in stored tissue blocks and preservation by cold storage of unstained slides. Am J Clin Pathol. 2017;148(5):398–415.
41. Vis AN, Kranse R, Nigg AL, van der Kwast TH. Quantitative analysis of the decay of immunoreactivity in stored prostate needle biopsy sections. Am J Clin Pathol. 2000;113(3):369–73.
42. Toubaji A, Sutcliffe S, Chaux A, et al. Immunohistochemical expression of minichromosome maintenance complex protein 2 predicts biochemical recurrence in prostate cancer: a tissue microarray and digital imaging analysis-based study of 428 cases. Hum Pathol. 2012;43(11):1852–65.
43. Gelb AB, Freeman VA, Astrow SH. Evaluation of methods for preserving PTEN antigenicity in stored paraffin sections. Appl Immunohistochem Mol Morphol. 2011;19(6):569–73.
44. Wester K, Wahlund E, Sundström C, et al. Paraffin section storage and immunohistochemistry. Effects of time, temperature, fixation, and retrieval protocol with emphasis on p53 protein and MIB1 antigen. Appl Immunohistochem Mol Morphol. 2000;8(1):61–70.
45. Quinn GP, Pentz RD, Muñoz-Antonia T, et al. Patient, caregiver and physician perspectives on participating in a thoracic rapid tissue donation program. Patient Educ Couns. 2018;101(4):703–10.
46. Baker JN, Windham JA, Hinds PS, et al. Bereaved parents' intentions and suggestions about research autopsies in children with lethal brain tumors. J Pediatr. 2013;163(2):581–6.
47. Weiner AB, Cortes-Mateus S, De Luis E, Durán I. Dural metastases in advanced prostate cancer: a case report and review of the literature. Curr Urol. 2013;7(3):166–8.
48. Spunt SL, Vargas SO, Coffin CM, et al. The clinical, research, and social value of autopsy after any cancer death: a perspective from the Children's Oncology Group Soft Tissue Sarcoma Committee. Cancer. 2012;118(12):3002–9.

Autopsy in the Twenty-First Century: Looking Forward

10

Jody E. Hooper

Introduction

The medical literature has forecast the ultimate end of the hospital autopsy numerous times in the past 40 years. The same reasons for its decline are cited repeatedly: lack of interest by pathologists, confidence in clinical diagnostic acumen, concerns about litigation, and perhaps most tellingly, lack of reimbursement. Despite these factors, the hospital autopsy continues to exist and in some settings is actually growing. The time has come to stop reexamining the past of the autopsy, cease ruminating on former glories, and look ahead to what hospital autopsy can become. Autopsy can demonstrate its value in an increasingly outcome-based medical system by growing and evolving as do all other modalities of diagnostic investigation. Furthermore, it can become an essential part of cutting-edge molecular research.

What Is Past and What Is to Come

Autopsy Has Been A modality for the elucidation of fundamental principles of disease.

Autopsy Can Become A continuing and expanding method for discovery of new disease entities.

The autopsy once was one of the most important means of discovery of the most fundamental principles of disease development, spread, and treatment. From the initial human anatomic descriptions by Herophilus in ancient Greece, through

J. E. Hooper
Department of Pathology, The Johns Hopkins University, Baltimore, MD, USA
e-mail: jhooper9@jhmi.edu

J. E. Hooper, A. K. Williamson (eds.), *Autopsy in the 21st Century*,
https://doi.org/10.1007/978-3-319-98373-8_10

becoming a key component of medical care with Morgagni during the Renaissance, the role of the autopsy has continuously evolved and changed. The correlations of morphologic observations and clinical events by Rokitansky opened the door to understanding of the multitude of diseases explicated by the autopsy in the twentieth century.

In our modern age of imaging and laboratory testing, however, the autopsy represents only one relatively non-technological modality for finding and exploring new pathologic processes. Even in this era, however, the autopsy brings unique assets to medical investigation. The autopsy provides a holistic view of the patient's disease through its comprehensive review of clinical/historical events and its physical examination (where permitted) of all organ systems. Autopsy brings a "helicopter-height" perspective which may not be available to caregivers during the patient's life, particularly in the current inpatient setting of multiple subspecialty consultants. Further, autopsy is an ideal tool for recognizing trends across individual patients and patient populations. For example, autopsy data on the high prevalence of incidental prostate cancer in older men played a major role in the recent discrediting of prostate-specific antigen testing (PSA) as a screening test [1]. This type of analytical insight does require the ability to compare results across patients, institutions, and regions, however, and the current divergent methods of performing and reporting autopsy do not lend themselves to harnessing the powerful data available in autopsies.

Autopsy Has Been Variably practiced and sporadically used for examination of diagnostic discrepancies.

Autopsy Can Become Characterized and supported by centers of excellence that establish national and international standards for diagnostic quality.

For autopsy to act as a genuine measure for quality assurance and quality control, fundamental changes in its practice may be necessary. Autopsy practitioners must not only have measures in place for evaluating the quality of their own work but should proactively pursue opportunities for participation in institutional quality management. Most programs provide some type of clinicopathologic correlation within reports, and they may present such findings at conferences; however, the missing step is ensuring that the data is used for system-wide change. Cases flagged for diagnostic discrepancies within a laboratory information system (LIS) and analyzed in conjunction with clinical colleagues should also be passed forward within the hospital quality management system. Unlike a medical record review alone, autopsy findings do not depend on input from a care team, and they lend objectivity to confirmation of diagnoses and discrepancy findings.

To fulfill their function as performance monitors that will encourage intervention to correct potential problems, autopsies must be performed in a sufficient quantity. The literature shows that physicians are often unable to accurately predict which cases will yield unexpected results [2]. *Improving Diagnosis in Health Care* by the

Institute of Medicine recently indicated that high-quality autopsies with standardized and easy-to-access data should be a part of data collection to assess current diagnostic accuracy [3]. The cost-effectiveness of autopsy's contribution to quality healthcare should be evaluated at least in part by its long-term and systemic benefits.

Autopsy Has Been Beautifully written prose descriptions which frequently are released after the opportunity for true clinical correlation has been lost, and the data is not retrievable or comparable across institutions.

Autopsy Can Become Prompt synoptic reporting integrated into more comprehensive laboratory information systems with data that can be electronically searched, retrieved, and compared across institutions.

Hill and Anderson's seminal text *The Autopsy and Public Policy* contains a priceless quote describing autopsy reports all too accurately: "every little thing along the way gets equal attention. And you write it all down in a voluminous report that is intelligible to very few people other than yourself and you send off 16 or 18 pages… to the patient's doctor who has no time to spend…trying to figure out the pathologists' language" [4]. The autopsy report must evolve for greater readability, with a focus on conciseness, and be promptly released if it is to demonstrate its value in the modern healthcare system.

Pre- and postmortem diagnostic discrepancies still exist, with major discrepancies that would have changed care management and perhaps affected survival persisting at rates of 5–8% [5, 6]. As yet, studies evaluating discrepancy rates are largely single institution and very often performed within a single medical subspecialty. Harnessing the vast stores of data within autopsies on a cross-institutional and national level is a tantalizing idea, but it will require autopsy reports to be structured with discrete data points that can be digitally retrieved en masse. Many institutions have created templates for autopsy gross descriptions, but it would be better still to have an accepted national standard which autopsy services around the country would utilize. Creativity and flexibility will be needed to address the question of how to modernize more complex sections of the autopsy report such as clinical history and diagnoses, but the benefits of standardized reporting to pathology departments, clinicians, researchers, and society would be enormous.

Autopsy Has Been An uncredited activity considered to be too costly in terms of time and money for many practitioners or small institutions to support.

Autopsy Can Become A regionalized activity that consistently demonstrates value in autopsy, is evaluated as part of pathologists' workloads, and proves essential to just and meaningful malpractice litigation.

Autopsy is not reimbursed by any type of medical insurance in the United States. This fact has much to do with a lack of enthusiasm for autopsy among pathologists, particularly those in private practice settings where autopsies are already relatively rare. The concept of a regionalized center for performance of autopsy is not new and has been implemented in many academic centers. Economies of scale will reduce costs for well-equipped regional centers, and pooling of expertise (and indeed enthusiasm) will increase quality of autopsy performance, reporting, and education. Several authors have proposed models for evaluating professional autopsy efforts using multiples of the current CPT coding system and incorporating them into wRVU calculations [7, 8]. However, even when such work assessments are not tied to any direct billing, the objective documentation and acknowledgment of work associated with autopsy performance is useful and will help convey the effort involved in the endeavor. Studies have shown that malpractice cases in which an autopsy was involved, including those in which diagnostic discrepancies were identified, do not correlate with unfavorable outcomes for the clinicians involved [9]. It is important that every autopsy be performed with the care and diligence that a pathologist would use in a known medicolegal case.

Autopsy Has Been Practiced in a traditional fashion with any additional testing driven by the background, interests, and ideas of individual autopsists.

Autopsy Can Become A flexible and nimble instrument with data-driven and universally supported protocols for special patient populations.

There are no nationally or internationally agreed-upon autopsy protocols either for special patient populations (the elderly, obese patients) or for particular disease processes (sepsis, congenital abnormalities). It is important for pathologists to be aware of the spectrum of findings in patients with disorders such as anorexia, bulimia, or anabolic steroid use as autopsy results and population findings in these disorders can influence public policy. Also, the collection and storage of ancillary testing specimens such as blood and tissue cultures, body fluids, and frozen tissue differ widely among institutions and regions.

Partly due to a lack of standardization in the performance of the autopsy itself, there is a paucity of data from which to draw conclusions about what specimens should be taken, at what time point, and in which patients. In keeping with the usual apprenticeship model of teaching, autopsy practice is largely a matter of the past experience, preferences, and interests of the individual practitioner. If truly data-driven retrospective studies prove too cumbersome to conduct, at least a pooling of collective experience to develop accepted standards is definitely needed.

Autopsy Has Been Iconoclastically taught by attending pathologists with varying degrees of investment in its principles, ideas, practices, and applications.

Autopsy Can Become Standardized applied learning of the integration of clinical, physical, and laboratory data and the teaching of principles of diagnosis and tissue handling applicable across pathologic specialties.

Autopsy teaching has historically been conducted by the apprenticeship model, but with numbers of cases decreasing and experienced mentors in shorter supply, this method is showing its flaws. The Association of Pathology Chairs Autopsy Working Group survey demonstrated that many programs currently have no Autopsy Service Director, and for others, there is little to no communication between the Autopsy Service Director and the Residency Director regarding fulfillment of program educational objectives. Genuine and systemic documentation of the competency of learners is needed. The concept of Entrustable Professional Activities (EPAs) is one alternative that has been considered. Although there has been much discussion about reducing the current required number of 50 autopsies for pathology residents, a majority of Autopsy Program Directors surveyed opined that the number was either "about right" or too few [10]. The Working Group also concluded that training must be improved and better standardization achieved before any consideration of reducing required autopsy numbers can be considered.

It is important to note that autopsy rotations teach far more than simply technical competency in anatomic dissection. Autopsy provides opportunities for holistic review of patient history, complex interpretation of clinician and family communication, decision-making regarding laboratory testing and consultation, and synthesis of all of these inputs into a comprehensive report. The skills it imparts will be highly useful and foundational even to a resident who never performs another autopsy after training.

Autopsy Has Been A method for discovery and explanation of the effects of criminal activity and an aid to its prosecution.

Autopsy Can Become A tool that uses sophisticated technology to help set public policy for wide-reaching disease and social epidemics.

Autopsy has developed through history not only as a method of medical discovery but as a tool for criminal investigation. In the modern world, forensic pathologists collect evidence, provide professional opinions and insights, interpret observations, and testify in criminal cases, but they can also fulfill wide-ranging general health functions such as identifying public health hazards, recognizing disease outbreaks, and monitoring for bioterrorism. It is worth noting that only about half of the US population resides in geographic areas covered by a Medical Examiner Office, with the other half living in areas covered by appointed or elected Coroners who are not necessarily medically trained. Systems vary even more widely internationally. The opioid crisis in particular has highlighted the fact that the forensic pathology specialty is chronically understaffed and underfunded.

The Consortium of Forensic Science Organizations (CFSO) is advocating for multiple measures including mandatory accreditation for ME/C offices, a federal office of forensic medicine, model state legislation for the establishment of medical examiner offices, and funding for operations, training, and research. With this type of support, medical examiner offices would be able to take advantage of technologies such as advanced imaging (CT or MRI), genetic testing, and proteomic analysis. Medical examiner roles could then also expand to encompass greater roles in public health, forensic medicine for the living, and biomedical research.

Autopsy Has Been Involved in retrospective and observational research resulting in a decline in numbers and impact of publications within the field.

Autopsy Can Become An integral part of clinical trials and cutting-edge cancer and other disease research and essential to the role of discovery in an era of systemic and heterogenous disease.

Autopsies are now being performed on an urgent basis to collect tumor and other tissues for researchers. Rapid autopsies, as they are called, can provide tissue specimens in large volumes and can sample across numerous anatomic sites simultaneously. Rapid autopsies also yield samples at a point in the patient's treatment course when it is usually impossible to obtain tissue for research due to the acuity of illness and invasiveness of biopsy or resection procedures. These autopsy specimens can also be compared with samples from earlier in the disease course. Autopsy specimens have proven capable of producing living cell lines and xenograft specimens and have yielded genetic sequencing and other study data. Studies utilizing rapid autopsy have led to the discovery of new genes associated with prostate cancer, characterized the pancreatic cancer exome, and supported the first profiling of the human proteome [11–13].

Most rapid research autopsy programs in the United States and internationally are associated with large academic centers. Key factors for development of a program include clearly delineating the scope of and relationship of the program with researchers, identifying participants, and arranging for logistics of death notification and transport. It is extremely important to have proper consenting for use of study tissue as well as for the autopsy procedure itself. The adherence to best collection practices during the autopsy can make the difference between usable and non-usable samples. Rapid autopsy represents a valued contribution by patients and families and an extraordinary avenue for autopsy to fulfill a new purpose.

Into the Twenty-First Century

Autopsy is enjoying an unusual moment in the public spotlight, thanks to its portrayal on television and other media. There is in some senses a greater interest in bringing the autopsy forward among the lay public than there is among medical professionals. Carrying the autopsy into the future will require constant education and demonstration of value to clinical and pathology colleagues. Autopsy practitioners must seek out and welcome new roles in informing public policy, contributing to patient safety, and embracing research and participation in clinical trials. If the autopsy can grow and change, mirroring broader transformations in the practice of pathology, science, and medicine, it can compete on its own merits. As with other medical subspecialties, the time may have come for an international consensus conference to set universally agreed-upon standards for the practice, reporting, and teaching of the autopsy.

The editors sincerely hope this book imparts knowledge, helps improve skills, and provides the inspiration needed for the autopsy to reassert its vital presence at the heart of medicine for the twenty-first century and beyond. The fate of this invaluable asset to clinical care, education, public policy, and research is up to all of us.

References

1. Bell KJL, Del Mar C, Wright G, et al. Prevalence of incidental prostate cancer: a systematic review of autopsy studies. Int J Cancer. 2015;137(7):1749–57.
2. Shojania KG, Burton EC, Goldman L. The autopsy as an outcome and performance measure. Evid Rep Technol Assess (Summ). 2002;58:1–5.
3. Institute of Medicine Committee on Diagnostic Error in Health Care. In: Balogh EP, Miller BT, editors. Improving Diagnosis in Health Care. Washington DC: National Academies Press; 2015.
4. Hill RE, Anderson RE. The autopsy – medical practice and public policy. 1st ed. Butterworth-Heinemann; 1988. Ebook 9781483192635.
5. Shojania KG, Burton EC, McDonald KM, et al. Changes in rates of autopsy detected diagnostic errors over time: a systematic review. JAMA. 2003;289:2849–56.
6. Goldman L, Sayson R, Robbins S, Cohn LH, Bettmann M, Weisberg M. The value of the autopsy in three medical eras. NEJM. 1982;301:1000–5.
7. Sinard JH, Autopsy Committee of the College of American Pathologists. Accounting for the professional work of pathologists performing autopsies. Arch Pathol Lab Med. 2013;137(2):228–32.
8. Taylor GP, Faye-Petersen OM, Ernst L, et al. Small patients, complex challenging cases: a reappraisal of the professional efforts in perinatal autopsies. Arch Pathol Lab Med. 2014;138(7):865–8.
9. Bove KE, Iery C, Autopsy Committee of the College of American Pathologists. The role of the autopsy in medical malpractice cases, I: a review of 99 appeals court decisions. Arch Pathol Lab Med. 2002;126(9):1023–31.
10. Davis GG, et al. Report and recommendations of the Association of Pathology Chairs' Autopsy Working Group. Manuscript in preparation.
11. Kibel AS, Schutte M, Kern SE, Isaacs WB, Bova GS. Identification of 12p as a region of frequent deletion in advanced prostate cancer. Cancer Res. 1998;58(24):5652–5.
12. Jones S, Zhang X, Parsons DW, Lin JC-H, Leary RJ, Angenendt P, Mankoo P, Carter H, Kamiyama H, Jimeno A, Hong S-M, Fu B, Lin M-T, Calhoun ES, Kamiyama M, Walter K, Nikolskaya T, Nikolsky Y, Hartigan J, Smith DR, Hidalgo M, Leach SD, Klein AP, Jaffee EM, Goggins M, Maitra A, Iacobuzio-Donahue C, Eshleman JR, Kern SE, Hruban RH, Karchin R, Papadopoulos N, Parmigiani G, Vogelstein B, Velculescu VE, Kinzler KW. Core signaling pathways in human pancreatic cancers revealed by global genomic analyses. Science. 2008;321(5897):1801–6. PMCID: PMC2848990.

13. Kim M-S, Pinto SM, Getnet D, Nirujogi RS, Manda SS, Chaerkady R, Madugundu AK, Kelkar DS, Isserlin R, Jain S, Thomas JK, Muthusamy B, Leal-Rojas P, Kumar P, Sahasrabuddhe NA, Balakrishnan L, Advani J, George B, Renuse S, Selvan LDN, Patil AH, Nanjappa V, Radhakrishnan A, Prasad S, Subbannayya T, Raju R, Kumar M, Sreenivasamurthy SK, Marimuthu A, Sathe GJ, Chavan S, Datta KK, Subbannayya Y, Sahu A, Yelamanchi SD, Jayaram S, Rajagopalan P, Sharma J, Murthy KR, Syed N, Goel R, Khan AA, Ahmad S, Dey G, Mudgal K, Chatterjee A, Huang T-C, Zhong J, Wu X, Shaw PG, et al. A draft map of the human proteome. Nature: Nature Publishing Group. 2014;509(7502):575–81. PMCID: PMC4403737.

Index

J. E. Hooper, A. K. Williamson (eds.), *Autopsy in the 21st Century*,
https://doi.org/10.1007/978-3-319-98373-8